Fourth Edition

Pocket Guide to Huszar's
BASIC DYSRHYTHMIAS
and Acute Coronary Syndromes

INTERPRETATION AND MANAGEMENT

Keith Wesley, MD

With 141 illustrations

Medical Director, HealthEast Medical Transportation, St. Paul, Minnesota
Medical Director, United EMS, Wisconsin Rapids, Wisconsin
Medical Director, Chippewa Fire District, Chippewa Falls, Wisconsin

ELSEVIER
MOSBY JEMS

3251 Riverport Lane
St. Louis, Missouri 63043

ISBN: 978-0-323-03973-4

Vice President and Publisher: Andrew Allen
Executive Editor: Linda Honeycutt Dickison
Senior Developmental Editor: Laura Bayless
Publishing Services Manager: Julie Eddy
Senior Project Manager: Andrea Campbell
Design Direction: Jessica Williams

Printed in China

Last digit is the print number: 9 8 7 6 5 4 3 2 1

This book is dedicated to my wife Karen, and three sons JT, Austin, and Camden.
Without your love, confidence, and patience, I could not have pursued my dream.

I love you.

It is with great gratitude and humility that I continue Dr. Huszar's legacy of this wonderful text

Keith Wesley, MD

About the Author

Keith Wesley is a board-certified emergency medicine physician living in Wisconsin. Originally from Tyler, Texas, he graduated from Brigham Young University in 1982 and Baylor College of Medicine in Houston Texas in 1986. He completed an Emergency Medicine Residency at Methodist Hospital in Indianapolis, Indiana, where he gained his first exposure to EMS, flying air medical missions.

Dr. Wesley has been involved in EMS since 1989, working with many services in Wisconsin. In 1992, he was selected by the Governor as a founding member of the Wisconsin State Physician Advisory Committee and served for 12 years, the last 4 years as Chair. In 2006, Dr. Wesley was selected as the Wisconsin State EMS Medical Director and continues to provide medical oversight to several services throughout Wisconsin.

From 1992 to 2004, Dr. Wesley was a Clinical Assistant Professor, University of Wisconsin Family Practice Residency, Eau Claire, Wisconsin responsible for the training and education of family practice residents rotating through the emergency department. During the same period, Dr. Wesley was an ACLS instructor overseeing the courses throughout south central Wisconsin.

In 2008, Dr. Wesley moved his practice to Minnesota when he accepted the position as the Minnesota State EMS Medical Director. He currently works for HealthEast Care Systems in St. Paul, where he is the EMS Medical Director for HealthEast Medical Transportation.

Dr. Wesley is a former chair of the National Council of State EMS Medical Directors and is active in the National Association of EMS Physicians. He has co-authored four textbooks and numerous articles and papers on EMS and is a frequent speaker at state and national EMS conferences. He is currently on the editorial board for *JEMS* magazine.

An active member of the American College of Emergency Physicians and the National Association of EMS Physicians, Dr. Wesley has been actively involved in the creation of educational programs for medical and nursing students, EMTs, and physicians.

When not engaged in EMS duties Dr. Wesley enjoys sailing on Lake Superior with his wife Karen and spending time with his three sons.

Author Acknowledgments

First, I would like to thank the dedicated men and women of my EMS services who provided me encouragement, criticism, and reams of rhythms strips and 12 leads. They include HealthEast Medical Transportation, Chippewa Fire District, Higgins Ambulance, and the EMT-Basic services of Ashland and Bayfield Counties.

Next, I must acknowledge the successful foundation upon which this book is based. Dr. Huszar expertly crafted this text in three previous editions. To be given the opportunity to carry on where this great man left off is an honor.

Finally, no author can accomplish anything without an editor. I have been most fortunate to have not one but two excellent editors with Laura Bayless and Andrea Campbell. Thank you both for the encouragement to make this project a success. Also, I'd like to thank Linda Honeycutt for giving me this opportunity and her endless support.

Publisher Acknowledgments

The editors wish to acknowledge the reviewers of the fourth edition of this book for their invaluable assistance in developing and fine-tuning this manuscript.

Janet Fitts, RN, BSN, CEN, TNS, EMT-P
Owner/Educational Consultant
    Prehospital Emergency Medical Education
    Pacific, Missouri
Paramedic/Training Officer
    New Haven Ambulance District
    New Haven, Missouri

Mark Goldstein, RN, MSN, EMT-P I/C
Emergency Services Operations Manager
Memorial Health System–Emergency & Trauma Center
Colorado Springs, Colorado

Kevin T Collopy, BA, CCEMT-P, NREMT-P, WEMT
Lead Instructor
    Wilderness Medical Associates
Flight Paramedic
    Spirit MTS, St. Joseph's Hospital
    Marshfield, Wisconsin

Robert L. Jackson, Jr., BA, MAPS, MAR, NREMT-P, CCEMT-P
Paramedic
University of Missouri Healthcare
Columbia, Missouri

Ronald N. Roth, MD, FACEP
Professor of Emergency Medicine
    University of Pittsburgh, School of Medicine
Medical Director, City of Pittsburgh
    Department of Public Safety
    Pittsburgh, Pennsylvania

Lynn Pierzchalski-Goldstein, PharmD
Clinical Coordinator
Penrose St. Francis Health System
Colorado Springs, Colorado

David L. Sullivan, PhD, NREMT-P
Program Director
Emergency Medical Services–Continuing Medical Education
St. Petersburg College–Health Education Center
Pinellas Park, Florida

Gilbert N. Taylor, FF/NREMT-P,I/C
Fire Investigator
Bourne Fire & Rescue
Bourne, Massachusetts

Our continued thanks also go out to the previous edition reviewers, whose hard work continues to contribute to the ongoing success of this book: Robert Carter, Robert Cook, Robert Elling, Timothy Frank, Glen A. Hoffman, Kevin B. Kraus, Mikel Rothenburg, Judith Ruple, Ronald D. Taylor, Glen Treankler, and Andrew W. Stern.

Preface

This text was written to teach medical, nursing, and EMS providers the basic skills in cardiac dysrhythmia interpretation. Once this is accomplished, the student discovers advanced instruction in the clinical signs, symptoms, and management of patients presenting with cardiac dysrhythmias.

With the advent of ECG monitoring has come readily accessible 12-lead electrocardiography, an essential tool in the detection and management of acute coronary syndromes. It is for that reason that this edition has added several chapters dedicated to 12-lead ECG interpretation. Following these, the student is provided an in-depth review of the pathophysiology, clinical signs and symptoms, and management of acute coronary syndromes.

The amount of anatomy, physiology, and pathophysiology has been significantly increased from the previous edition to better enable the student to develop a more comprehensive understanding of the cause of particular dysrhythmias and coronary syndromes. This knowledge provides the student additional tools to accurately interpret and manage the presented dysrhythmias and conditions.

Each dysrhythmia is presented in its "classic," form with an associated table listing its unique characteristics. These tables can be used as a quick reference. The accompanying text contains a more detailed and extensive discussion of these characteristics.

The vast majority of rhythm strips are from real patients and will not always include all of the "classic" characteristics described in the text. This is the challenge of ECG dysrhythmia interpretation and the student should take this into consideration when examining any rhythm strip.

The treatment algorithms are based on the latest information from the American Heart Association and the American College of Cardiology recommendations. However, because the science continues to evolve and local policy and protocol may vary, the student should remain abreast of new treatments and consult local medical experts to ensure that their treatment remains current.

Keith Wesley, MD

The author and publisher have made every attempt to check dosages and advanced life support content for accuracy. The care procedures presented here represent accepted practices in the United States. They are not offered as a standard of care. Advanced life support–level emergency care is performed under the authority of a licensed physician. It is the student's responsibility to know and follow local care protocols as provided by his or her medical advisors. It is also the student's responsibility to stay informed of emergency care procedure changes, including the most recent guidelines set forth by the American Heart Association and printed in their textbooks.

Contents

1 ECG Fundamentals

Anatomy of the Heart

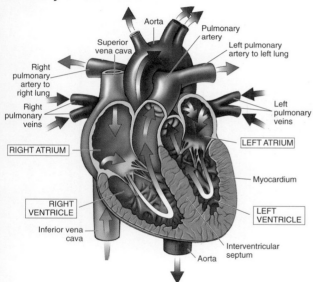

Conduction System of the Heart

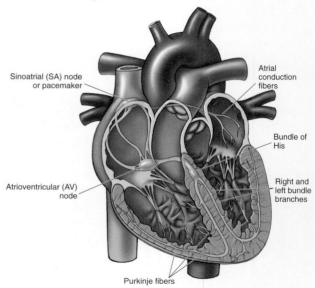

Coronary Circulation

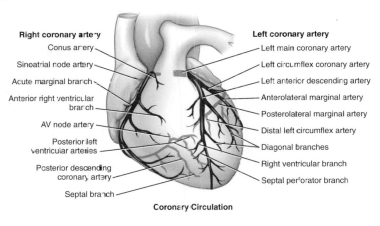

Right coronary artery
- Conus artery
- Sinoatrial node artery
- Acute marginal branch
- Anterior right ventricular branch
- AV node artery
- Posterior left ventricular arteries
- Posterior descending coronary artery
- Septal branch

Left coronary artery
- Left main coronary artery
- Left circumflex coronary artery
- Left anterior descending artery
- Anterolateral marginal artery
- Posterolateral marginal artery
- Distal left circumflex artery
- Diagonal branches
- Right ventricular branch
- Septal perforator branch

Coronary Circulation

ECG Monitoring Leads

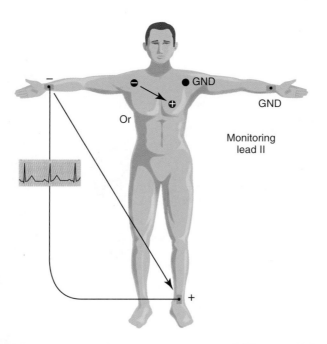

GND

GND

Or

Monitoring
lead II

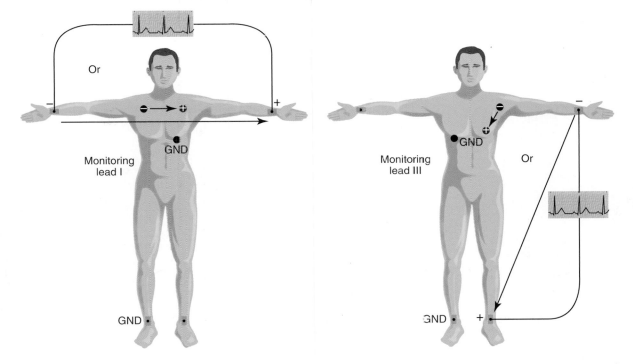

Or

Monitoring
lead I

GND

GND

Or

Monitoring
lead III

GND

GND

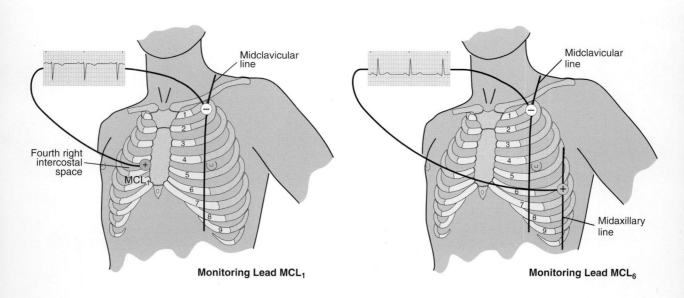

Monitoring Lead MCL₁

Monitoring Lead MCL₆

The 12-Lead ECG

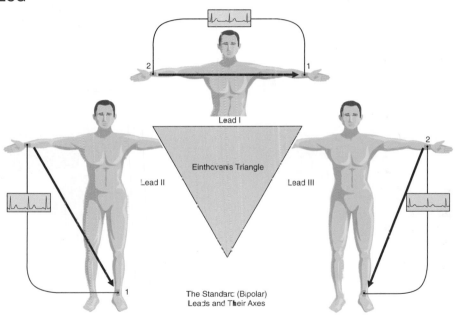

Einthoven's Triangle

Lead I

Lead II   Lead III

The Standard (Bipolar)
Leads and Their Axes

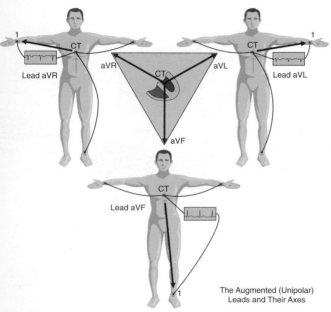

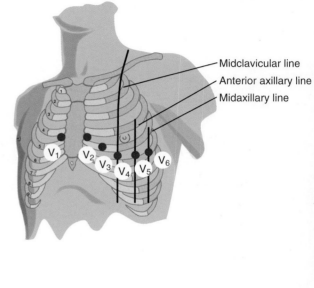

Midclavicular line

Anterior axillary line

Midaxillary line

The Augmented (Unipolar)
Leads and Their Axes

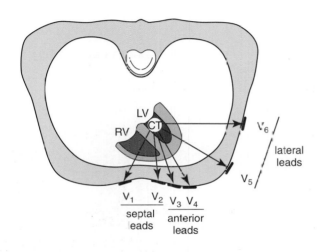

The Precordial Lead Axes

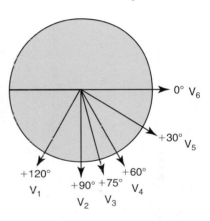

Precordial Reference Figure

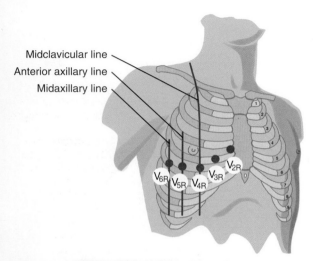

Midclavicular line

Anterior axillary line

Midaxillary line

Right-Sided Chest Leads

Components of the Electrocardiogram
Waves
P Wave

QRS Complex

T Wave

U Wave

Intervals
QT interval

R-R interval

Segments
ST segment

PR segment

WAVES

P Wave
Normal Sinus P Wave

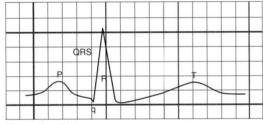

Normal Sinus P Wave

Significance: Represents normal depolarization of the right and left atria, which proceeds from right to left and downward.

ECG Characteristics

Direction: Positive (upright) in lead II.
Duration: 0.10 second or less.
Amplitude: 0.5 to 2.5 mm in lead II.
Shape: Smooth and rounded.
P Wave–QRS Complex Relationship: Each normally followed by a QRS complex; exception: atrioventricular (AV) block.
PR Interval: May be normal (0.12 to 0.20 second) or abnormal (greater than 0.20 second or less than 0.12 second).
Origin Site: Sinoatrial (SA) node.

Abnormal Sinus P Wave

II

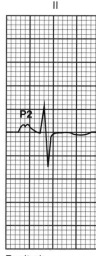

II

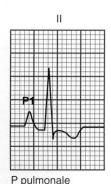

P pulmonale   P mitrale

Significance: Represents depolarization of altered, damaged, or abnormal atria, which proceeds from right to left and downward. Abnormal sinus P waves may be seen in the following:

- Increased right atrial pressure and right atrial dilatation and hypertrophy (right atrial overload) resulting from chronic obstructive pulmonary disease (COPD), status asthmaticus, acute pulmonary embolism, and acute pulmonary edema (tall and symmetrically peaked P waves [**P pulmonale**] in leads II, III, and aVF; biphasic P waves in leads V_1-V_2)
- Sinus tachycardia (abnormally tall P waves)
- Increased left atrial pressure and left atrial dilatation and hypertrophy (left atrial overload) resulting from hypertension, mitral and aortic valvular disease, acute myocardial infarction (MI), and pulmonary edema secondary to left-sided heart failure (wide, notched P waves [**P mitrale**] in leads I, II, and V_4-V_6; biphasic P waves in leads V_1-V_2)
- Delay or block of the progression of electrical impulses through the interatrial conduction tract between the right and left atria (wide, notched P waves [**P mitrale**])

Origin Site: SA node.

ECG Characteristics

Direction: Positive (upright) in lead II.

Duration: May be normal (0.10 second or less) or greater than 0.10 second.

Amplitude: May be normal (0.5 to 2.5 mm) or greater than 2.5 mm in lead II. A P pulmonale is 2.5 mm or greater in amplitude.

Shape: May be tall and symmetrically peaked (P pulmonale) or wide and notched (P mitrale). The P waves may be biphasic in leads V_1 and V_2.

P Wave–QRS Complex Relationship: Each normally followed by a QRS complex; exception: AV block.

PR Interval: May be normal (0.12 to 0.20 second) or abnormal (greater than 0.20 second or less than 0.12 second).

Ectopic P Wave (P Prime or P′)

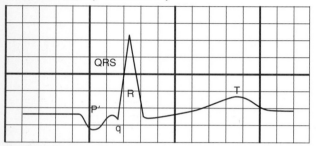

Ectopic P Wave (P Prime or P′)

Significance: Represents abnormal atrial depolarization occurring in an abnormal direction or sequence or both, the direction and sequence depending on the ectopic pacemaker's location.
- If the ectopic pacemaker is in the upper or middle part of the right atrium, depolarization of the atria occurs in a normal direction (right to left and downward).
- If the ectopic pacemaker is in the lower part of the right atrium near the AV node or in the left atrium or if it is in the AV junction or the ventricles, in which case the electrical impulse travels upward through the AV junction into the atria (retrograde conduction), the atria depolarize from left to right and upward (retrograde atrial depolarization).

Ectopic P waves occur in various atrial, junctional, and ventricular dysrhythmias, including the following:
- Wandering atrial pacemaker
- Premature atrial contractions
- Atrial tachycardia
- Premature junctional contractions
- Junctional escape rhythm
- Nonparoxysmal junctional tachycardia
- Paroxysmal supraventricular tachycardia
- Premature ventricular contractions (occasionally)

Origin Site: An ectopic pacemaker in the atria outside of the SA node or in the AV junction or ventricles.

ECG Characteristics
Direction:
- Positive (upright) in lead II, often resembling a normal sinus P wave, if the ectopic pacemaker is in the upper or middle right atrium
- Negative (inverted) in lead II if the ectopic pacemaker is in the lower right atrium near the AV node or in the left atrium, AV junction, or ventricles

Duration: 0.10 second or less or greater than 0.10 second.

Amplitude: Usually less than 2.5 mm in lead II, but may be greater.

Shape: May be smooth and rounded, peaked, or slightly notched.

P Wave–QRS Complex Relationship: May precede, be buried in, or follow the QRS complex with which it is associated.

P′R/RP′ Interval: Relationship between site of ectopic pacemaker, type of interval, and duration:

- Upper or middle part of the right atrium: P′R interval normal (0.12 to 0.20 second)
- Lower part of the atria, close to the AV node: P′R interval slightly less than 0.12 second
- Upper part of the AV junction: P′R interval less than 0.12 second
- Lower part of the AV junction or in the ventricles: RP′ interval usually less than 0.21 second

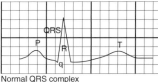

Normal QRS complex

QRS Complex

Normal QRS Complex

Significance: Represents normal depolarization of the right and left ventricles, which begins with the depolarization of the interventricular septum from left to right, producing the Q wave, and then continues with the depolarization of the ventricles from the endocardium to the epicardium, producing the R and S waves.

Origin Site: The SA node or an ectopic or escape pacemaker in the atria or AV junction.

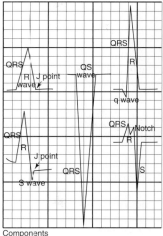

Components

ECG Characteristics

Components: The QRS complex consists of one or more of the following positive (upright) deflections (the R waves) and negative (inverted) deflections (the Q, S, and QS waves):

- **Q wave:** The first negative deflection in the QRS complex not preceded by an R wave.
- **R wave:** The first positive deflection in the QRS complex. Subsequent positive deflections that extend above the baseline are called *R prime (R′)*, *R double prime (R″)*, and so forth.
- **S wave:** The first negative deflection that extends below the baseline in the QRS complex following an R wave. Subsequent negative deflections are called *S prime (S′)*, *S double prime (S″)*, and so forth.
- **QS wave:** A QRS complex that consists entirely of a single, large negative deflection.

Note: Although there may be only one Q wave, there can be more than one R and S wave in the QRS complex.

- **Notch:** A notch in the R wave is a negative deflection that does not extend below the baseline; a notch in the S wave is a positive deflection that does not extend above the baseline.

The large waves that form the major deflections are identified by uppercase letters **(QS, R, S).** The smaller waves that are less than one-half the amplitude of the major deflections are identified by lowercase letters **(q, r, s).** Thus the ventricular depolarization complex can be described more accurately by using uppercase and lowercase letters assigned to the waves (e.g., **qR, Rs, qRs**).

Direction: May be predominantly positive (upright), predominantly negative (inverted), or equiphasic (equally positive, equally negative).

Duration:

- QRS complex: 0.12 second or less (0.06 to 0.12 second) in adults and 0.08 second or less in children.
- Q wave: 0.04 second or less.

Ventricular Activation Time (VAT): The time from the onset of the QRS complex to the peak of the R wave; normally 0.05 second or less, but may be greater than 0.05 second in left ventricular hypertrophy.

Amplitude: The amplitude of the R or S wave in the QRS complex in lead II may vary from 1 to 2 mm to 15 mm or more. The normal Q wave is less than 25% of the height of the succeeding R wave.

Shape: The QRS complex waves are generally narrow and sharply pointed.

Junction (J) Point: The end of the QRS complex at the point where the QRS complex becomes the ST segment.

Abnormal QRS Complex

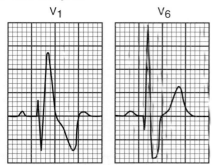

Right bundle branch

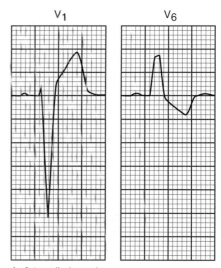

Left bundle branch

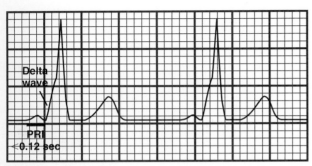

Ventricular Preexcitation

Significance: Represents abnormal depolarization of the ventricles, which may result from one of the following:

- **Intraventricular conduction disturbance.** The most common forms are right and left bundle branch block; a less common form, a nonspecific, diffuse intraventricular conduction defect (IVCD), is seen in MI, fibrosis, and hypertrophy; electrolyte imbalance, such as hypokalemia and hyperkalemia; and excessive administration of such cardiac drugs as quinidine, procainamide, and flecainide. May be seen in supraventricular rhythms and dysrhythmias.
- **Aberrant ventricular conduction (aberrancy).** A temporary delay in the conduction of an electrical impulse through the bundle branches usually caused by the premature appearance of the electrical impulse at the bundle branches while they are still partially refractory and unable to conduct normally. The result is an abnormally wide QRS complex that often resembles an incomplete or complete bundle branch block. Aberrancy is most commonly seen in premature atrial and junctional complexes and supraventricular tachydysrhythmias.

- **Ventricular preexcitation.** Premature depolarization of the ventricles caused by abnormal conduction of electrical impulses from the atria or AV junction to the ventricles via an accessory conduction pathway (the accessory AV pathway) bypassing the AV junction—the classic form of ventricular preexcitation. The result is a shorter than normal PR interval (0.09 to 0.12 sec) and a wide QRS complex (0.10 sec or more) with an initial slurring of the upward slope of the R wave (or of the downstroke of the S wave, as the case may be)—the *delta wave*. Another preexcitation syndrome, the *nodoventricular/fasciculoventricular preexcitation,* involving an accessory conduction pathway between the lower part of the AV node or the bundle of His and the ventricles, also results in an abnormally wide QRS complex with a delta wave but with a normal PR interval.
- **Ventricular dysrhythmias.** Dysrhythmias that originate in an ectopic ventricular or escape pacemaker located in the bundle branches, Purkinje network, or ventricular myocardium.

ECG Characteristics

Components: The same as in normal QRS complexes. In addition, if ventricular preexcitation is present, an initial delta wave is usually present.

Direction: May be predominantly positive (upright), predominantly negative (inverted), or equiphasic (equally positive, equally negative).

Duration: Greater than 0.12 second.

Amplitude: Varies from 1 to 2 mm to 20 mm or more.

Shape: Varies widely in shape, from one that appears quite normal—narrow and sharply pointed (as in incomplete bundle branch block and aberrant ventricular conduction and in ventricular dysrhythmias arising in the bundle branches)—to one that is wide and bizarre, slurred and notched (as in complete bundle branch block and aberrant ventricular conduction and in ventricular dysrhythmias arising in the Purkinje network and ventricular myocardium).

T Wave

Normal T Wave

Significance: Represents normal repolarization of the ventricles, which proceeds from the epicardium to the endocardium.

ECG Characteristics

Direction: Positive (upright) in lead II.
Duration: 0.10 to 0.25 second or greater.
Amplitude: Less than 5 mm in standard leads.
Shape: Sharply or bluntly rounded and slightly asymmetrical, the first, upward part being longer than the second, downward part.
T Wave–QRS Complex Relationship: Always follows the QRS complex.

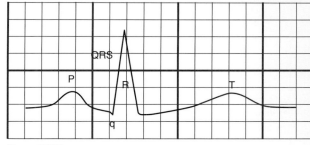

Normal T Wave

Abnormal T Wave

Significance: Represents abnormal ventricular repolarization, which may proceed (a) from the epicardium to the endocardium as it normally does, but at a slower rate than usual, producing an abnormally tall, upright T wave in lead II, or (b) from the endocardium to the epicardium, producing a negative T wave in lead II. Abnormal ventricular repolarization may occur in the following:

- Myocardial ischemia, acute MI, myocarditis, pericarditis
- Ventricular enlargement (hypertrophy)
- Electrolyte imbalance (e.g., excess serum potassium)
- Administration of certain cardiac drugs (e.g., quinidine, procainamide)
- Bundle branch block and ectopic ventricular dysrhythmias
- In athletes and in persons who are hyperventilating

ECG Characteristics

Direction: May be positive (upright) and abnormally tall or low, negative (inverted), or biphasic (partially positive and partially negative) in lead II. The abnormal T wave may or may not be in the same direction as that of the normal QRS complex. The T wave following an abnormal QRS complex is usually in the opposite direction of it and abnormally wide and tall, is usually deflected in the opposite direction of the QRS complex, and is abnormally wide and tall.

Duration: 0.10 to 0.25 second or greater.

Amplitude: Variable.

Shape: May be rounded, blunt, sharply peaked, wide, or notched.

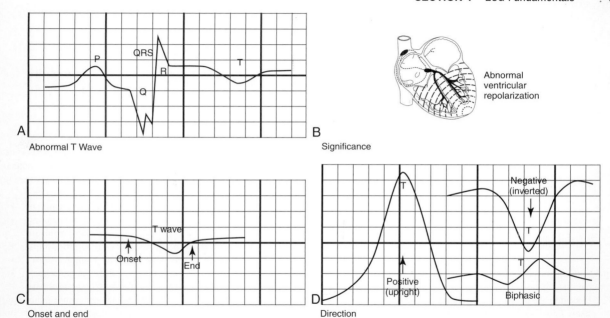

A Abnormal T Wave

B Significance

Abnormal ventricular repolarization

C Onset and end

D Direction

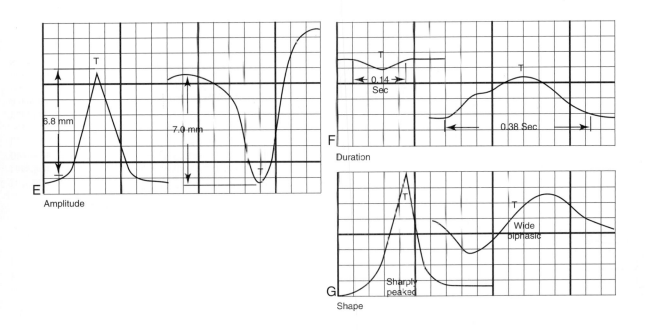

E

Amplitude

F

Duration

G

Shape

U Wave

Significance: Probably represents the final stage of repolarization of a small segment of the ventricles (such as the papillary muscles or ventricular septum) after most of the right and left ventricles have been repolarized. Abnormally tall U waves may be present in the following:

- Hypokalemia
- Cardiomyopathy, left ventricular hypertrophy
- Excessive administration of digitalis, quinidine, procainamide, and amiodarone

ECG Characteristics

Location: On the downward slope of the T wave or following it.
Direction: Normally positive (upright), the same direction as that of the preceding normal T wave in lead II. Abnormal U waves may be positive (upright) or negative (inverted).
Duration: Usually not determined.
Amplitude: Normally less than 2 mm and always smaller than that of the preceding T wave in lead II. A U wave taller than 2 mm or the preceding T wave is considered to be abnormal.
Shape: Rounded and symmetrical.

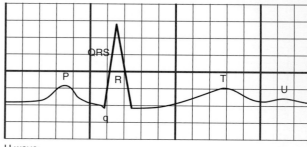

U wave

INTERVALS

QT Interval

Normal QT Interval

Significance: Represents the time between the onset of depolarization and the end of repolarization of the ventricles (i.e., the refractory period of the ventricles) and indicates that ventricular repolarization is normal.

ECG Characteristics

Onset and End: Begins with the onset of the QRS complex and ends with the end of the T wave.

Duration: Dependent on the heart rate, being shorter when the heart rate is fast and longer when the heart rate is slow. Normally, the QT interval is somewhat less than half of the preceding R-R interval; one that is greater than half is abnormal, and one that is approximately half is "borderline." The QT intervals may be equal or unequal in duration depending on the underlying rhythm. The average duration of the QT interval normally expected at a given heart rate is called the corrected QT interval (or QTc). The QTc plus or minus 10% values are shown in the table to the right. Regardless of the heart rate, a QT interval of greater than 0.45 second is considered abnormal.

QTc Intervals

Heart Rate (beats/min)	R-R Interval (sec)	QTc and Normal Range (sec)
40	1.5	0.46 (0.41-0.51)
50	1.2	0.42 (0.38-0.46)
60	1.0	0.39 (0.35-0.43)
70	0.86	0.37 (0.33-0.41)
80	0.75	0.35 (0.32-0.39)
90	0.67	0.33 (0.30-0.36)
100	0.60	0.31 (0.28-0.34)
120	0.50	0.29 (0.26-0.32)
150	0.40	0.25 (0.23-0.28)
180	0.33	0.23 (0.21-0.25)
200	0.30	0.22 (0.20-0.24)

Note: The determination of the QT interval should be made in the lead where the T wave is most prominent and not deformed by a U wave and should not include the U wave. Furthermore, the measurement of the QT interval assumes that the duration of the QRS complex is normal with an average value of 0.08 second. If the QRS is widened beyond 0.08 second for any reason, the excess widening beyond 0.08 second must be subtracted from the actual measurement to obtain the correct QT interval.

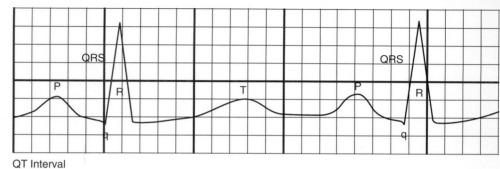

QT Interval

Abnormal QT Interval

Significance: Represents an abnormal rate of ventricular repolarization, either slower or more rapid than normal. An abnormally prolonged QT interval, one that exceeds the average QT interval for any given heart rate by 10%, indicates slowing of ventricular repolarization. This can occur in the following:

- Electrolyte imbalance (hypokalemia and hypocalcemia)
- Excess of certain drugs (e.g., quinidine, procainamide, disopyramide, amiodarone, phenothiazines, tricyclic antidepressants). The prolongation of the QT interval following administration of excessive amounts of such antidysrhythmic agents as quinidine, procainamide and disopyramide may provoke the appearance of torsade de pointes.
- Liquid protein diets
- Pericarditis, acute myocarditis, acute MI, and left ventricular hypertrophy
- Hypothermia
- Central nervous system disorders (e.g., cerebrovascular accident [CVA], subarachnoid hemorrhage, intracranial trauma)

- Without a known cause (idiopathic)
- Bradydysrhythmias (e.g., marked sinus bradycardia, third-degree AV block with slow ventricular escape rhythm)

An abnormally short QT interval, one that is less than the average QT interval (QTc) for any given heart rate by 10%, represents an increase in the rate of repolarization of the ventricles. This can occur in the following:

- Digitalis therapy
- Hypercalcemia

ECG Characteristics

Onset and End: The same as those of a normal PR interval.

Duration: Greater or less than the QTc for any given heart rate by 10%. A QT interval of greater than 0.45 second is considered abnormal regardless of the heart rate.

R-R Interval

Significance: Represents the time between two successive ventricular depolarizations during which the atria and ventricles contract and relax once (i.e., one cardiac cycle).

ECG Characteristics
Onset and End: Begins with the peak of one R wave and ends with the peak of the succeeding R wave.

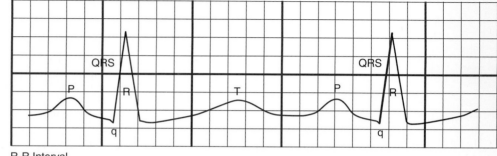

R-R Interval

Duration: Dependent on the heart rate, being shorter when the heart rate is fast and longer when the heart rate is slow (e.g., heart rate 120, R-R interval 0.50 second; heart rate 60, R-R interval 1.0 second). The R-R intervals may be equal or unequal in duration depending on the underlying rhythm.

PR Interval

Normal PR Interval

Significance: Represents the time from the onset of atrial depolarization to the onset of ventricular depolarization, during which the electrical impulse progresses normally and without delay from the SA node or an ectopic pacemaker in the atria through the electrical conduction system to the ventricular myocardium. The PR interval includes the P wave and PR segment.

Onset and End: Begins with the onset of the P wave and ends with the onset of the QRS complex.

Duration: Varies from 0.12 to 0.20 second, depending on the heart rate. Normally, it is shorter when the heart rate is fast and longer when the heart rate is slow (e.g., heart rate 120, PR interval 0.12 second; heart rate 60, PR interval 0.16 second).

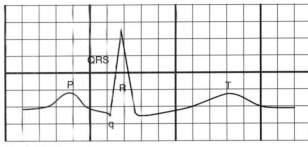

Normal PR Interval

Abnormal PR Interval

Significance: Represents the abnormal progression of the electrical impulse from the SA node or an ectopic or escape supraventricular pacemaker through the electrical conduction system to the ventricular myocardium. It may be greater than 0.20 second or less than 0.12 second.

- When greater than 0.20 second, it represents delayed progression of the electrical impulse through the AV node, bundle of His, or rarely, the bundle branches—AV block.
- When less than 0.12 second, it represents either of the following:
  (a) The origination of the electrical impulse in an ectopic pacemaker in the atria close to the AV node or in an ectopic or escape pacemaker in the AV junction; in both instances the P waves are commonly negative (inverted) in lead II.
  (b) The abnormal progression of the electrical impulse from the atria to the ventricles through an accessory conduction pathway that bypasses either the AV junction via the accessory AV pathway *(ventricular preexcitation)* or the AV node alone via the atrio-His fibers *(atrio-His preexcitation).* The P waves in these preexcitation syndromes are usually positive (upright) in lead II. The QRS complexes in ventricular preexcitation are abnormally wide, with a delta wave; those in atrio-His preexcitation are normal.

ECG Characteristics

Onset and End: The same as those of a normal PR interval.

Duration: May be greater than 0.20 second or less than 0.12 second.

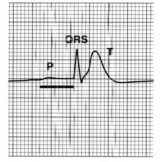

Abnormally Prolonged PR Interval

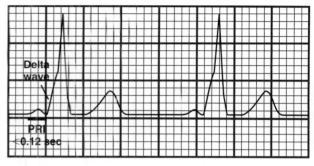

Abnormally Short PR Interval

SEGMENTS

ST Segment
Normal ST Segment
Significance: Represents the early part of normal repolarization of the right and left ventricles.

ECG Characteristics
Onset and End: Begins with the end of the QRS complex, the "junction" or "J" point, and ends with the onset of the T wave.
Duration: 0.20 second or less, depending on the heart rate, being shorter when the heart rate is fast and longer when the heart rate is slow.
Amplitude: Normally flat (isoelectric), but may be slightly elevated or depressed by less than 1.0 mm, 0.04 second (1 small square) after the J point of the QRS complex and still be normal.
Appearance: If slightly elevated, may be flat, concave, or arched. If slightly depressed, may be flat, upsloping, or downsloping.

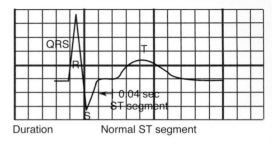

Duration   Normal ST segment

Abnormal ST Segment
Significance: Represents the early part of abnormal repolarization of the right and left ventricles, a common consequence of myocardial ischemia and acute MI, pericarditis, and hypothermia. It is also present in ventricular fibrosis and aneurysm, left ventricular hypertrophy, and administration of digitalis. ST-segment elevation may also occur normally as "early repolarization."

Onset and End: Same as those of a normal ST segment.

Duration: 0.20 second or less, depending on the heart rate, being shorter when the heart rate is fast and longer when the heart rate is slow.

Amplitude: Elevated or depressed 1.0 mm or more, 0.04 second (1 small square) after the J point of the QRS complex.

Appearance: If elevated, may be flat, concave, or arched. If depressed, may be flat, upsloping, or downsloping.

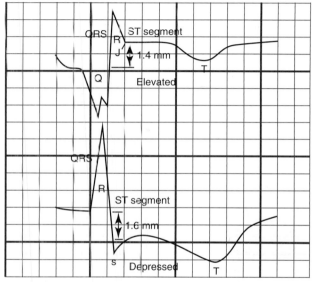

Amplitude   Abnormal ST segment

PR Segment

Significance: Represents the time from the end of atrial depolarization to the onset of ventricular depolarization during which the electrical impulse progresses from the AV node through the bundle of His, bundle branches, and Purkinje network to the ventricular myocardium.

ECG Characteristics

Onset and End: Begins with the end of the P wave and ends with the onset of the QRS complex.

Duration: Normally varies from approximately 0.02 to 0.10 second, but may be greater than 0.10 second if there is a delay in the progression of the electrical impulse through the AV node, bundle of His, or rarely, the bundle branches.

Amplitude: Normally, flat (isoelectric).

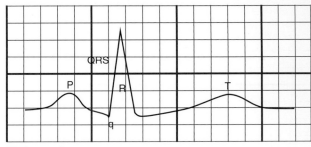

PR Segment

Normal ECG Components

P Waves: Normally, each followed by a QRS complex.
Direction: Positive (upright) in leads I, II, aVF, and V_4-V_6. Negative (inverted) in lead aVR. Positive, negative, or diphasic in leads III, aVL, and V_1-V_3.
Duration: 0.10 second or less.
Amplitude: 0.5 to 2.5 mm in lead II.
Shape: Smooth and rounded.

QRS Complexes: 0.12 second or less with generally narrow and sharply pointed waves.
Q Waves: 0.04 second or less in duration and less than 25% of the height of the succeeding R wave.
Ventricular Activation Time (VAT): 0.05 second or less

T Waves: Amplitude less than 5 mm in the standard limb and unipolar leads; less than 10 mm in the precordial leads.

PR Intervals: 0.12 to 0.20 second.

QT Intervals: Less than half the preceding R-R interval.

ST Segments: Flat, but may be elevated or depressed by no more than 1.0 mm, 0.04 second (1 small square) after the J point.

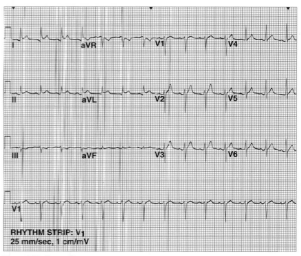

Normal Electrocardiogram

The ECG Lead Axes

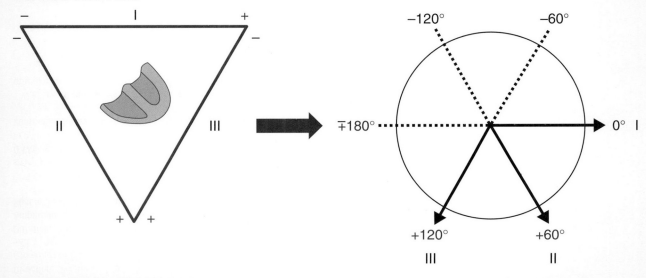

**Einthoven's Equilateral Triangle
Based on Leads I, II, and III**

**Triaxial Reference Figure
for Leads I, II, and III**

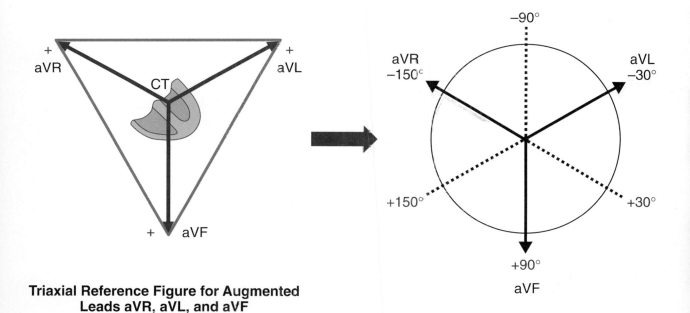

Triaxial Reference Figure for Augmented Leads aVR, aVL, and aVF

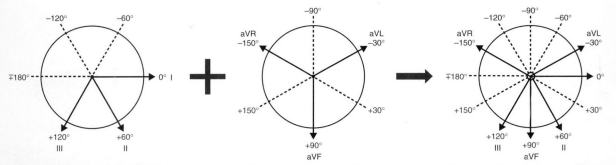

**Triaxial Reference Figure
Leads I, II, and III**

**Triaxial Reference Figure
Leads aVR, aVL, and aVF**

Hexaxial Reference Figure

The Three-Lead Method of Determining the QRS Axis

The three-lead method uses leads I, II, and aVF, and sometimes aVR in certain circumstances, to determine the general position of the QRS axis and to identify left and right axis deviation quickly.

Determine the net positivity or negativity of the QRS complexes in leads I, aVF, and II, in that order, as well as aVR if lead I is negative.

If lead I is *positive* and:

A. Leads aVF and II are predominantly positive, the QRS axis is between 0° and +90°.
B. Lead aVF is predominantly negative and lead II is predominantly positive, the QRS axis is between 0° and −30°.
C. Lead aVF is predominantly negative and lead II is equiphasic, the QRS axis is exactly −30°.
D. Leads aVF and II are predominantly negative, the QRS axis is between −30° and −90°.

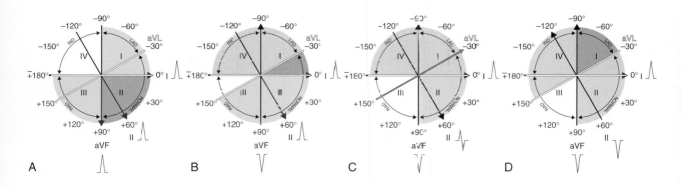

If lead I is *equiphasic* and:

E. Leads aVF and II are predominantly negative, the QRS axis is exactly −90°.

F. Leads aVF and II are predominantly positive, the QRS axis is exactly +90°.

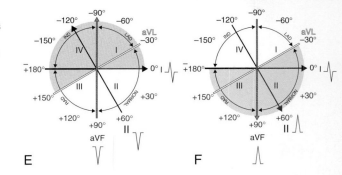

If lead I is *negative* and:

G(1). Leads aVF and II are predominantly positive, the QRS axis is between +90° and +150°.

G(2). If, in addition, lead aVR is also predominantly positive, the QRS axis is between +120° and +150°.

H. Lead aVF is predominantly positive and lead II is equiphasic, the QRS axis is exactly +150°.

I. Leads aVF and II are predominantly negative, the QRS axis is between −90° and −180°.

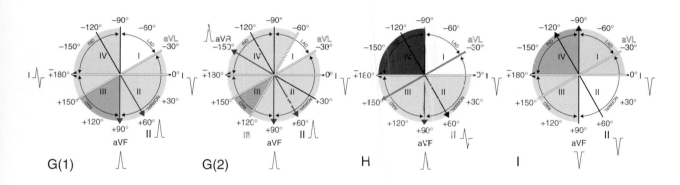

Summary of Three-Step Method

Figure	I	aVF	II	aVR	Location of QRS Axis
A	+	+	+		0° to +90°
B	+	−	+		0° to −30°
C	+	−	±		−30°
D	+	−	−		−30° to −90°
E	±	−	−		−90°
F	±	+	+		+90°
G(1)	−	+	+		+90° to +150°
G(2)	−	+	+	+	+120° to +150°
H	−	+	±		+150°
I	−	−	−		−90° to −180°

+, Predominantly positive; −, predominantly negative; ±, equiphasic.

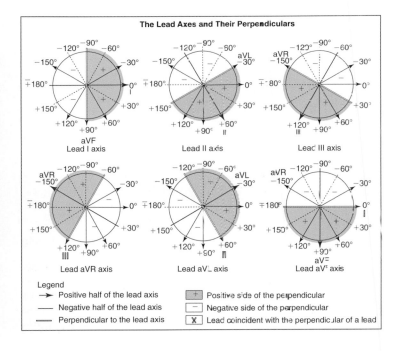

The Lead Axes and Their Perpendiculars

aVF
Lead I axis

Lead II axis

Lead III axis

Lead aVR axis

Lead aVL axis

Lead aVF axis

Legend
→ Positive half of the lead axis
— Negative half of the lead axis
— Perpendicular to the lead axis

[+] Positive side of the perpendicular
[−] Negative side of the perpendicular
[X] Lead coincident with the perpendicular of a lead

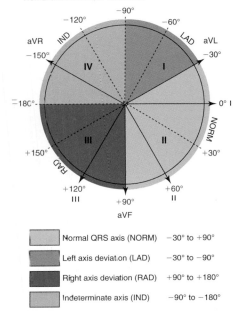

Normal and Abnormal QRS axes

Normal QRS axis (NORM)	−30° to +90°
Left axis deviation (LAD)	−30° to −90°
Right axis deviation (RAD)	+90° to +180°
Indeterminate axis (IND)	−90° to −180°

Eight Steps to ECG Interpretation

The following is an outline of the steps in interpreting an ECG to determine the presence of a dysrhythmia and its identity. The ECG interpretation may be performed in the order shown or in accordance with local prehospital or hospital protocols.

Dysrhythmia Determination

Step One: Determine the heart rate.

Step Two: Determine the regularity of the rhythm.

1. Classify as regular, regularly irregular, totally irregular.

Step Three: Identify and analyze the P, P′, F, or f waves.
1. Identify the P, P′, F, or f waves.
2. Determine the atrial rate and rhythm.
3. Note the relationship of the P, P′, F, or f waves to the QRS complexes.

Step Four: Determine the PR or RP′ intervals and AV conduction ratio.

1. Determine the PR (or RP′) intervals.
2. Assess the equality of the PR (or RP′) intervals.
3. Determine the AV conduction ratio.

Step Five: Identify and analyze the QRS complexes.
1. Identify the QRS complexes.
2. Note the duration and shape of the QRS complexes.
3. Assess the equality of the QRS complexes.

Step Six: Determine the site of origin of the dysrhythmia.

Step Seven: Identify the dysrhythmia.

Step Eight: Evaluate the clinical significance of the dysrhythmia. The following is an outline of the steps in interpreting a 12-lead ECG to determine the presence of an acute coronary syndrome. The ECG interpretation may be performed in the order shown or in accordance with local prehospital or hospital protocols.

Acute Coronary Syndrome Identification

Step One: Identify any abnormally elevated or depressed ST segments and the leads where noted.

Step Two: Identify any abnormally tall or inverted T waves and the leads where noted.

Step Three: Identify any Q waves and the leads where noted.

Step Four: Identify any abnormally tall, diminished, or absent R waves and the leads where noted.

Step Five: Based on the above analysis, determine the following in the figure:
1. The presence and location of ischemia, injury, or infarction.

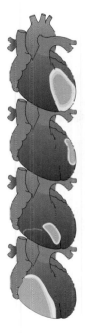

Surface of the Heart Viewed	Facing Leads
Anterior	V_1-V_4
Lateral	I, aVL, V_5-V_6
Inferior	II, III, aVF
Right ventricle	V_{4R}

Dysrhythmia Identification

Normal Sinus Rhythm (NSR)

Rate: 60 to 100 beats/min.

Regularity: Essentially regular.

P Waves: Upright in lead II; identical and precede each QRS complex.

PR Intervals: Normal (0.12 to 0.20 second); constant.

R-R Intervals: Equal.

QRS Complexes: Usually normal (0.12 second or less), unless a preexisting intraventricular conduction delay is present.

Site of Origin: SA node.

Treatment: None.

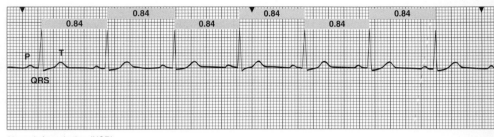

Normal Sinus Rhythm

Normal sinus rhythm (NSR)

The most common form of intraventricular conduction delay is a right or left bundle branch block. A less common form is a nonspecific, intraventricular conduction defect (IVCD) seen in myocardial infarction (MI), fibrosis, and hypertrophy; electrolyte imbalance, such as hypokalemia and hyperkalemia; and excessive administration of such cardiac drugs as quinidine and procainamide.

Sinus Dysrhythmia

Rate: 60 to 100 beats/min. Typically, the heart rate increases during inspiration and decreases during expiration.

Regularity: Regularly irregular.

P Waves: Upright in lead II; identical and precede each QRS complex.

PR Intervals: Normal (0.12 to 0.20 second); constant.

R-R Intervals: Unequal; shorter during inspiration, longer during expiration.

QRS Complexes: Usually normal (0.12 second or less), unless a preexisting intraventricular conduction delay is present.

Site of Origin: SA node.

Treatment: None.

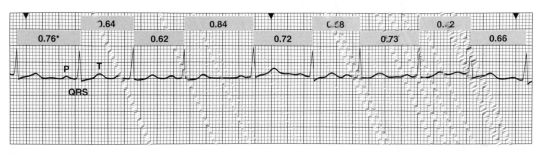

Sinus dysrhythmia

Sinus Bradycardia

Rate: Less than 60 beats/min.

Regularity: Essentially regular.

P Waves: Upright in lead II; identical and precede each QRS complex.

PR Intervals: Normal (0.12 to 0.20 second); constant.

R-R Intervals: Equal.

QRS Complexes: Usually normal (0.12 second or less), unless a preexisting intraventricular conduction delay is present.

Site of Origin: SA node.

Treatment: See Section III, page 94.

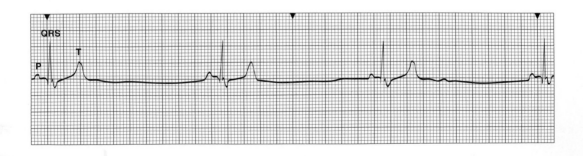

Sinus Arrest and Sinoatrial (SA) Exit Block

Rate: 60 to 100 beats/min or less.

Regularity: Irregular when sinus arrest or SA exit block is present.

P Waves: Absent when sinus arrest or SA exit block is present (dropped P wave).

PR Intervals: Absent when sinus arrest or SA exit block is present.

R-R Intervals: Unequal when sinus arrest or SA exit block is present.

QRS Complexes: Usually normal (0.12 second or less), unless a preexisting intraventricular conduction delay is present.

Site of Origin: SA node.

Treatment: See Section III, page 94.

Sinus Arrest and Sinoatrial Exit Block

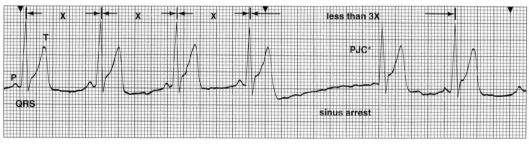

Sinus arrest

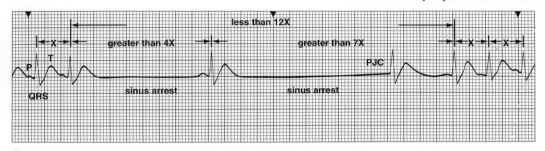

Sinus arrest

Sinus Tachycardia

Rate: More than 100 beats/min, can be as high as 180 beats/min.

Regularity: Essentially regular.

P Waves: Normal, or slightly taller and more peaked than normal; upright in lead II; identical and precede each QRS complex.

PR Intervals: Normal (0.12 to 0.20 second); constant.

R-R Intervals: Usually equal, but may be slightly unequal.

QRS Complexes: Usually normal (0.12 second or less), unless a preexisting intraventricular conduction delay or aberrant ventricular conduction is present.

Site of Origin: SA node.

Treatment: No specific treatment indicated. See Section III, page 97. A temporary delay in the conduction of an electrical impulse through the bundle branches producing an abnormally wide QRS complex, caused by the arrival of the electrical impulse at the bundle branches prematurely while they are still partially refractory and unable to conduct normally. The QRS complex may show a right or left bundle branch block pattern or a combination of a right bundle branch block pattern and a left anterior or posterior fascicular block pattern.

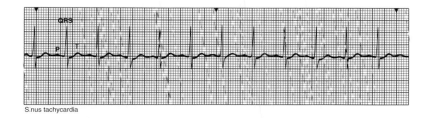

Sinus tachycardia

Wandering Atrial Pacemaker (WAP)

Heart Rate: Usually 60 to 100 beats/min, but may be less.

Regularity: Usually irregular.

P Waves: Gradually change in size, shape, and direction from normal,

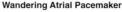
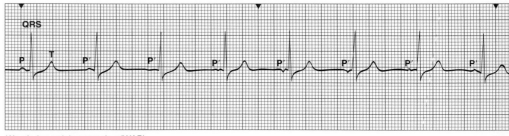
Wandering atrial pacemaker (WAP)

positive (upright) P waves to abnormally small, even negative (inverted) P′ waves over a series of beats, and then back again to normal in a reverse sequence; precede each QRS complex.

PR Intervals: Unequal; varies within normal limits (0.12 to 0.20 second) from approximately 0.20 second to approximately 0.12 second over a series of beats.

R-R Intervals: Usually unequal.

QRS Complexes: Usually normal (0.12 second or less), unless a preexisting intraventricular conduction delay is present.

Site of Origin: Shifts back and forth between the SA node and an ectopic pacemaker in the atria or atrioventricular (AV) junction.

Treatment: No specific treatment indicated.

Premature Atrial Complexes (PACs)

Rate: That of the underlying rhythm.

Regularity: Irregular when PACs are present.

P' Waves: P' waves occur earlier than the next expected P sinus. The size, shape, and direction of the P' waves depend on the location of the pacemaker site. P' waves followed by QRS complexes related to them are *conducted* PACs. P' waves occurring alone, not followed by QRS complexes, are *nonconducted, dropped,* or *blocked* PACs.

P-P Intervals: The P-P' interval (coupling interval) is usually shorter, and the P'-P interval is the same or slightly longer than the P-P interval of the underlying rhythm. Commonly, a non-compensatory pause is present (i.e., the sum of the P-P' and the P'-P intervals is less than twice the P-P interval of the underlying rhythm). Rarely, a compensatory pause is present (i.e., the sum of the P-P' and the P'-P intervals is equal to twice the underlying P-P interval).

P'R Intervals: Normal (0.12 to 0.20 second); may vary between PACs.

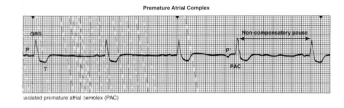

Premature Atrial Complex

isolated premature atrial complex (PAC)

R-R Intervals: Unequal when PACs are present.

QRS Complexes: Usually normal (0.12 second or less), resembling those of the underlying rhythm. If aberrant ventricular conduction is present, the PAC may be wide and bizarre, resembling a premature ventricular contraction (PVC)—PAC with aberrancy.

Site of Origin: An ectopic pacemaker in the atria.

Treatment: See Section III, page 111.

Types of PACs

Infrequent PACs: Less than five PACs/min.

Frequent PACs: Five or more PACs/min.

Isolated PACs (Beats): PACs occurring singly.

Group Beats: PACs occurring in groups of two or more.

Paired PACs (Couplet): Two PACs in a row.

Atrial Tachycardia: Three or more PACs in a row.

Atrial Bigeminy: PACs alternating with the QRS complexes of the underlying rhythm.

Atrial Trigeminy/Atrial Quadrigeminy: PACs following every two or three QRS complexes of the underlying rhythm, respectively.

Lead II

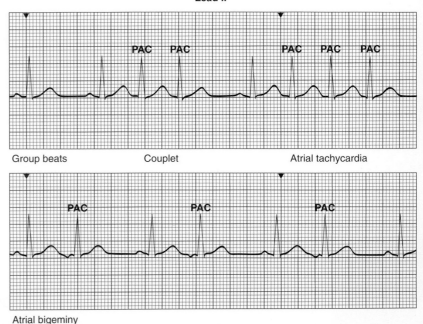

Group beats   Couplet   Atrial tachycardia

Atrial bigeminy

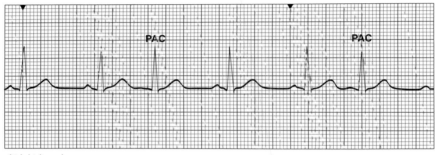

Atrial trigeminy

Atrial Tachycardia (Ectopic Atrial Tachycardia, Multifocal Atrial Tachycardia [MAT])

Rate: Usually 160 to 240 beats/min.

Regularity: Essentially regular. Onset and termination are usually gradual.

P′ Waves: The P′ waves, which usually precede the QRS complexes, may be either: (1) positive (upright) in lead II if they originate in the atria near the SA node or (2) negative (inverted) if they originate in the atria near the AV junction. The P′ waves are usually identical in any given lead in ectopic atrial tachycardia, but in MAT they vary in size, shape, and direction in each given lead. When P′ waves are not always followed by a QRS complex, atrial tachycardia with block is present (e.g., a 2:1, 3:1, or 4:1 block). The P′ waves are often buried in the preceding T or U waves or QRS complexes.

P′R Intervals: The P′R intervals are usually normal (0.12 to 0.20 second) and constant in ectopic atrial tachycardia; in MAT they vary slightly from 0.20 second to less than 0.12 second in each given lead.

R-R Intervals: Usually equal in ectopic atrial tachycardia without block, but will vary in MAT. The R-R intervals will also vary in atrial tachycardia with block.

QRS Complexes: Usually normal (0.12 second or less), unless a preexisting intraventricular conduction delay, aberrant ventricular conduction, or ventricular preexcitation is present. If the wide and bizarre QRS complexes occur only with the atrial tachycardia, the dysrhythmia is called *atrial tachycardia with aberrancy* (or *atrial tachycardia with aberrant ventricular conduction*). Such a tachycardia usually resembles ventricular tachycardia.

Site of Origin: An ectopic pacemaker in the atria. When a single ectopic pacemaker site is present, the dysrhythmia is called *ectopic atrial tachycardia;* when three or more pacemaker sites are present, it is called *multifocal atrial tachycardia (MAT).*

Treatment: See Section III, pages 98-99.

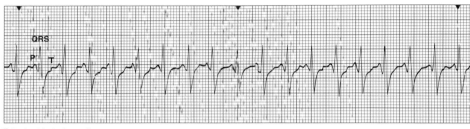

Ectopic atrial tachycardia

Abnormal conduction of electrical impulses from the atria to the ventricles via an accessory AV pathway bypassing the AV junction and causing premature activation of the ventricles. This commonly results in a shorter than normal PR interval (0.09 to 0.12 second) and a wide QRS complex (greater than 0.12 second) with an initial slurring of the upward slope of the R wave (the delta wave).

Atrial Flutter

Rate: Atrial rate: 240 to 360 (average, 300) F waves/min. Ventricular rate: Usually approximately 150 beats/min if atrial flutter is uncontrolled (untreated); 60 to 75 beats/min if controlled (treated) or if a preexisting AV block is present.

Regularity: Usually regular, but may be irregular.

F Waves: Sawtooth-shaped repetitive waves.

FR Intervals: Usually equal, but may be unequal.

R-R Intervals: Usually equal and constant, but may be unequal.

QRS Complexes: Usually normal (0.12 second or less), unless a preexisting intraventricular conduction delay, aberrant ventricular conduction, or ventricular preexcitation is present.

Site of Origin: An ectopic pacemaker in the atria.

Treatment: See Section III, pages 103-105.

Atrial Flutter

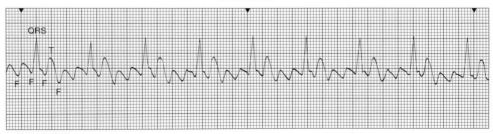

Atrial flutter (4:1)

Atrial Fibrillation (AF)

Rate: Atrial rate: 350 to 600 or more (average, 400) f waves/min.

Ventricular Rate: Usually 160 to 180 beats/min if atrial fibrillation is uncontrolled (untreated); 60 to 70 beats/min if controlled (treated) or if a preexisting AV block is present.

Regularity: Totally irregular.

f Waves: Irregularly shaped, rounded (or pointed), and dissimilar atrial fibrillation (f) waves. If the f waves are large (≥1 mm), "coarse" fibrillatory waves are present; if they are small (<1 mm), "fine" fibrillatory waves are present.

P-R Intervals: None.

R-R Intervals: Typically unequal.

QRS Complexes: Usually normal (0.12 second or less), unless a preexisting intraventricular conduction delay, aberrant ventricular conduction, or ventricular preexcitation is present.

Site of Origin: Multiple ectopic pacemakers in the atria.

Treatment: See Section III, pages 103-105.

Atrial Fibrillation

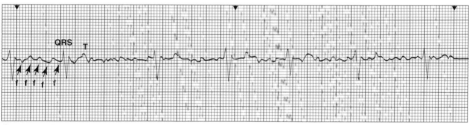

Coarse atrial fibrillation

Junctional Escape Rhythm

Rate: 40 to 60 beats/min, but may be less.

Regularity: Essentially regular.

P′ Waves: P waves may be present or absent. If present, they either (1) regularly precede or follow each QRS complex, in which case they are negative (inverted) in lead II having originated in the AV junction (P′ waves), or (2) occur independently, being either positive (upright) or negative (inverted) in lead II. If the P waves occur independently of the QRS complexes, AV dissociation is present. The pacemaker site of such P waves is the SA node or an ectopic pacemaker in the atria.

P′R/RP′ Intervals: If the P′ waves regularly precede the QRS complexes, the P′R intervals are abnormal (less than 0.12 second). If the P′ waves regularly follow the QRS complexes, the RP′ intervals are less than 0.20 second.

R-R Intervals: Usually equal.

QRS Complexes: Usually normal (0.12 second or less), unless a preexisting intraventricular conduction delay is present.

Site of Origin: An escape pacemaker in the AV junction.

Treatment: See Section III, page 96.

Junctional Escape Rhythm

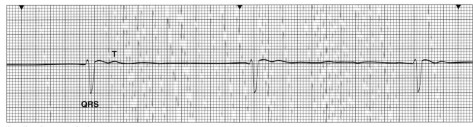

Junctional escape rhythm

Premature Junctional Complexes (PJCs)

Rate: That of the underlying rhythm.

Regularity: Irregular when PJCs are present.

P′ Waves: P′ waves may or may not be associated with the PJCs. If present, they usually differ from the P waves of the underlying rhythm in size, shape, and direction. The P′ waves are negative (inverted) in lead II. They may precede, be buried in, or less commonly, follow the QRS complexes of the PJCs. P′ waves followed or preceded by QRS complexes related to them are *conducted* PJCs; those occurring alone, not followed or preceded by QRS complexes, are *nonconducted* or *blocked* PJCs.

P′R/RP′ Intervals: If P′ waves regularly precede the QRS complexes of the PJCs, the P′R intervals are abnormal (less than 0.12 second). If P′ waves regularly follow the QRS complexes, the RP′ intervals are less than 0.20 second.

R-R Intervals: Unequal when PJCs are present. The pre-PJC R-R interval is shorter and the post-PJC R-R interval is longer than the R-R interval of the underlying rhythm. Commonly, a compensatory pause is present (i.e., the sum of the pre- and post-PJC R-R intervals is twice the R-R interval of the underlying rhythm). When the sum is less than twice the R-R interval of the underlying rhythm (uncommonly), a non-compensatory pause is present.

QRS Complexes: The QRS complexes of the PJCs occur earlier than the next expected QRS complex of the underlying rhythm. Usually, they are normal (0.12 second or less), resembling those of the underlying rhythm. If aberrant ventricular conduction is present, the PJC may be wide and bizarre, resembling a PVC—PJC with aberrancy.

Site of Origin: An ectopic pacemaker in the AV junction.

Treatment: See Section III, page 111.

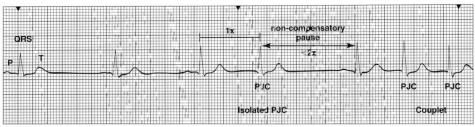

Premature Junctional Complexes

Premature junctional complexes (PJCs)

Types of PJCs

Infrequent PJCs: Less than five PJCs/min.

Frequent PJCs: Five or more PJCs/min.

Isolated PJCs (Beats): PJCs occurring singly.

Group Beats: PJCs occurring in groups of two or more.

Paired PJCs (Couplet): Two PJCs in a row.

Junctional Tachycardia: Three or more PJCs in a row.

Junctional Bigeminy: PJCs alternating with the QRS complexes of the underlying rhythm.

Junctional Trigeminy/Quadrigeminy: PJCs following every two or three QRS complexes of the underlying rhythm, respectively.

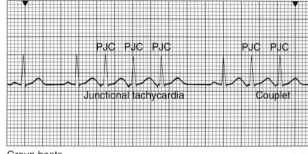

Group beats

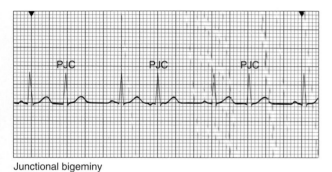

Junctional bigeminy

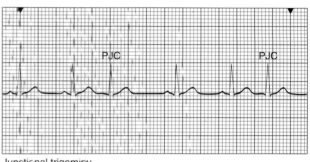

Junctional trigeminy

Nonparoxysmal Junctional Tachycardia (Accelerated Junctional Rhythm, Junctional Tachycardia)

Rate: Usually 60 to 130 beats/min, but may be as high as 150 beats/min. Accelerated junctional rhythm: 60 to 100 beats/min. Junctional tachycardia: 100 beats/min or greater. Onset and termination are usually gradual.

Regularity: Essentially regular.

P Waves: P waves may be present or absent. If present, they either (1) regularly precede or follow each QRS complex, in which case they are negative (inverted) in lead II, having originated in the AV junction (P′ waves), or (2) occur independently, being either positive (upright) or negative (inverted) in lead II. If the P waves occur independently of the QRS complexes, AV dissociation is present. The pacemaker site of such P waves is the SA node or an ectopic pacemaker in the atria.

P′R/RP′ Intervals: If P′ waves regularly precede the QRS complexes, the P′R intervals are abnormal (less than 0.12 second). If P′ waves regularly follow the QRS complexes, the RP′ intervals are less than 0.20 second.

R-R Intervals: Usually equal.

QRS Complexes: Usually normal (0.12 second or less), unless a preexisting intraventricular conduction delay or an aberrant ventricular conduction is present.

Site of Origin: An ectopic pacemaker in the AV junction.

Treatment: No specific treatment indicated.

Nonparoxysmal Junctional Tachycardia
(Accelerated Junctional Rhythm, Junctional Tachycardia)

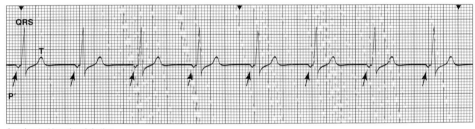

Accelerated junctional rhythm

Paroxysmal Supraventricular Tachycardia (PSVT)

Rate: Usually 160 to 240 beats/min. PSVT occurs in paroxysms, beginning abruptly and lasting a few seconds to many hours.

Regularity: Essentially regular.

P′ Waves: Present or absent. When present, the P′ waves usually follow the QRS complexes; rarely, they precede the QRS complexes. The P′ waves are generally negative (inverted) in lead II.

P′R Intervals: If the P′ waves precede each QRS complex, the P′R intervals are abnormal (less than 0.12 second). If the P′ waves follow each QRS complex, the RP′ intervals are less than 0.20 second. The P′R and RP′ intervals are usually constant.

R-R Intervals: Usually equal.

QRS Complexes: Usually normal (0.12 second or less), unless a preexisting intraventricular conduction delay or an aberrant ventricular conduction is present. If the wide and bizarre QRS complexes occur only with the PSVT, the dysrhythmia is called *PSVT with aberrancy* (or *PSVT with aberrant ventricular conduction*). Such a PSVT may resemble ventricular tachycardia.

Site of Origin: A reentry mechanism in the AV junction involving the AV node alone (AV nodal reentry tachycardia [AVNRT]) or the AV node and an accessory conduction pathway (AV reentry tachycardia [AVRT]).

Treatment: See Section III, page 101.

Paroxysmal Supraventricular Tachycardia

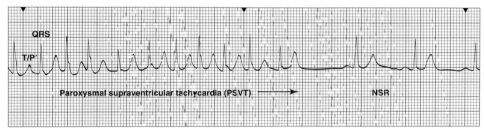

Ventricular Escape Rhythm

Rate: Usually 30 to 40 beats/min, but may be less.

Regularity: Regular, but may be irregular.

P Waves: P waves may be present or absent. If present, they usually bear no relation to the QRS complexes, marching between and through them. Such P waves originate in the SA node or an ectopic pacemaker in the atria or AV junction.

P'R/RP' Intervals: None.

R-R Intervals: Usually equal, but may be slightly unequal.

QRS Complexes: Typically wide (greater than 0.12 second) and bizarre. Usually identical, but may vary slightly.

Site of Origin: An escape pacemaker in the ventricles.

Treatment: See Section III, page 96.

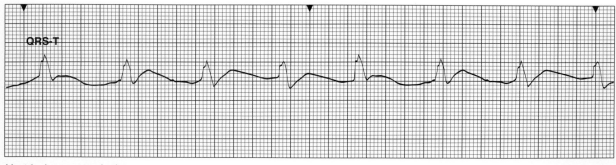

Ventricular escape rhythm

Accelerated Idioventricular Rhythm (AIVR)

Rate: 40 to 100 beats/min.

Regularity: Regular, but may be irregular.

P Waves: P waves may be present or absent. If present, they usually bear no relation to the QRS complexes, occurring independently of the QRS complexes. Such P waves originate in the SA node or an ectopic pacemaker in the atria or AV junction.

RP' Intervals: Present if the P' waves are associated with the PVCs, typically following them, usually less than 0.12 second.

R-R Intervals: Usually equal, but may be slightly unequal.

QRS Complexes: Typically wide (greater than 0.12 second) and bizarre. Usually identical, but may vary slightly.

Site of Origin: An ectopic pacemaker in the ventricles.

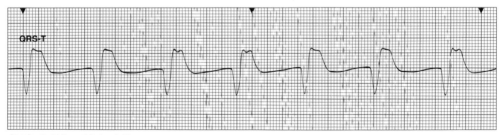

Accelerated idioventricular rhythm

Premature Ventricular Complexes (PVCs)

Rate: That of the underlying rhythm.

Regularity: Irregular when PVCs are present.

P Waves: P waves may be present or absent. If present, they are usually of the underlying rhythm and bear no relation to the PVCs, sometimes appearing as notches in the ST segment or T wave of the PVCs. Uncommonly, the P′ waves are related to the PVCs, in which case they follow the QRS complexes of the PVCs, appearing as negative (inverted) P′ waves or notches in the ST segments or T waves of the PVCs in lead II.

RP′ Intervals: Present if the P′ waves are associated with the PVCs, typically following them; approximately 0.20 second.

R-R Intervals: Unequal when PVCs are present. The coupling interval, the interval between the PVC and the preceding QRS complex of the underlying rhythm, is shorter and the post-PVC R-R interval is longer than the R-R interval of the underlying rhythm. Commonly, a complete compensatory pause is present (i.e., the sum of the coupling interval and the post-PVC R-R interval is twice the R-R interval of the underlying rhythm). Rarely, when the sum is less than twice the R-R interval of the underlying rhythm, an incomplete compensatory pause is present.

QRS Complexes: Typically wide (greater than 0.12 second) and bizarre. Identical PVCs are called *uniform PVCs*. PVCs with different QRS complexes are called *multiform PVCs*. PVCs with the same coupling intervals, indicating a single pacemaker site, are called *unifocal PVCs;* those with varying coupling intervals, indicating two or more pacemaker sites, are called *multifocal PVCs*. Usually, uniform PVCs are unifocal, whereas multiform PVCs are multifocal but can be unifocal.

Site of Origin: An ectopic pacemaker in the ventricles.

Treatment: See Section III, page 112.

Premature ventricular complexes

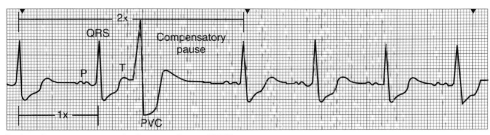

Isolated premature ventricular complexes (PVC)

Types of PVCs

Infrequent PVCs: Less than five PVCs/min.

Frequent PVCs: Five or more PVCs/min.

Isolated PVCs (Beats): PVCs occurring singly.

Paired PVCs (Couplet): Two PVCs in a row.

Ventricular Tachycardia: Three or more PVCs in a row.

Ventricular Bigeminy: PVCs alternating with the QRS complexes of the underlying rhythm.

Ventricular Trigeminy/Ventricular Quadrigeminy: PVCs following every two or three QRS complexes of the underlying rhythm, respectively.

R-on-T Phenomenon: A PVC occurring during the downslope of the preceding T wave (vulnerable period of ventricular repolarization).

Various Forms of PVCs

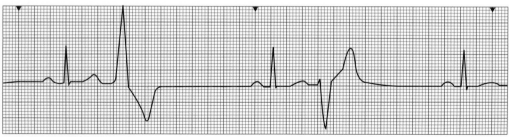

Multifocal PVCs: More than one shape

Lead II

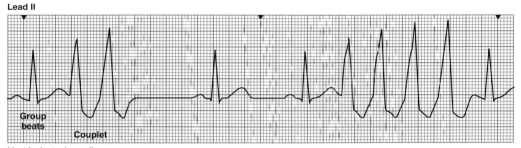

Ventricular tachycardia

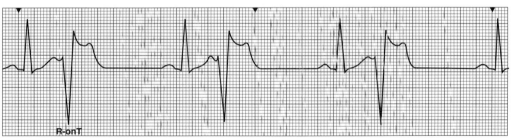

Ventricular bigeminy

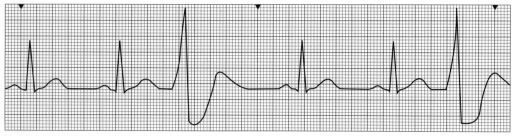

Ventricular trigeminy

Ventricular Tachycardia (VT)

Rate: Usually 110 to 250 beats/min.

Regularity: Usually regular, but may be slightly irregular.

P Waves: P waves may be present or absent. If present, they usually bear no relation to the QRS complexes, sometimes appearing here and there as notches in and between the ventricular complexes of the VT. Such P waves originate in the SA node or an ectopic pacemaker in the atria or AV junction. Uncommonly, the P′ waves are related to the VT, in which case they regularly appear as negative (inverted) P′ waves or notches in the latter part of the ventricular complexes or between them in lead II.

RP′ Intervals: Present if P′ waves regularly follow the QRS complexes; approximately 0.20 second.

R-R Intervals: Usually equal, but may be slightly unequal.

QRS Complexes: Typically wide (greater than 0.12 second) and bizarre. Usually identical, but may vary slightly *(monomorphic VT)*. Two distinctly different QRS complexes alternating with each other indicate a bidirectional VT. When the QRS complexes vary greatly, *polymorphic VT* is present. When the QRS complexes gradually change back and forth from one shape and direction to another over a series of beats, the VT is called *torsades de pointes*.

Site of Origin: An ectopic pacemaker in the ventricles.

Treatment: See Section III, pages 107-110.

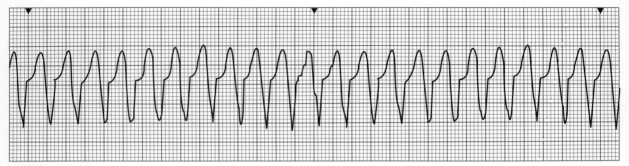

Ventricular tachycardia

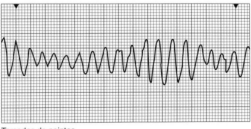

Torsades de pointes

Ventricular Fibrillation (VF)

Rate: 300 to 500 beats/min.

Regularity: Totally irregular.

P Waves: None.

PR Intervals: None.

R-R Intervals: None.

QRS Complexes: Irregularly shaped, rounded (or pointed), and significantly dissimilar fibrillation (f) waves. If the f waves are large (>3 mm), *coarse VF* is present; if the f waves are small (<3 mm), *fine VF* is present.

Site of Origin: Multiple ectopic pacemakers in the ventricles.

Treatment: See Section III, page 113.

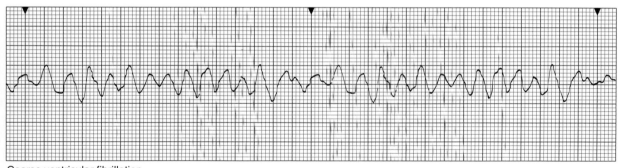

Coarse ventricular fibrillation

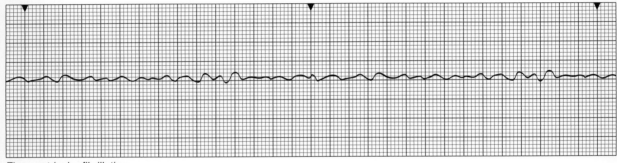

Fine ventricular fibrillation

Asystole

Rate: None.

Regularity: None.

P Waves: P waves may be present or absent.

PR Intervals: None.

R-R Intervals: None.

QRS Complexes: None.

Site of Origin: None.

Treatment: See Section III, page 114.

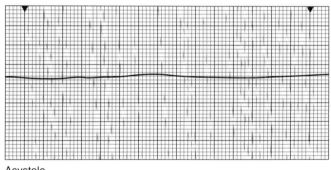

Asystole

First-Degree AV Block

First-Degree AV Block

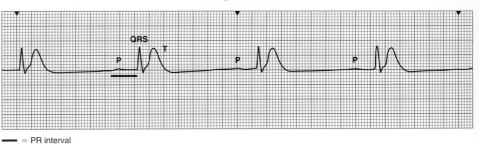

= PR interval

Rate: The atrial and ventricular rates are typically the same.

Regularity: That of the underlying rhythm.

P Waves: Those of the underlying rhythm; usually a QRS complex follows each P wave.

PR Intervals: Abnormal (greater than 0.20 second); usually do not vary from beat to beat.

R-R Intervals: Those of the underlying rhythm.

QRS Complexes: Usually normal (0.12 second or less), unless a preexisting intraventricular conduction delay is present.

AV Conduction Ratio: The AV conduction ratio is 1:1.

Treatment: No specific treatment indicated.

Second-Degree AV Block, Type I AV Block (Wenckebach)

Rate: The atrial rate is that of the underlying rhythm. The ventricular rate is typically less than the atrial rate.

Regularity: Patterned irregularity.

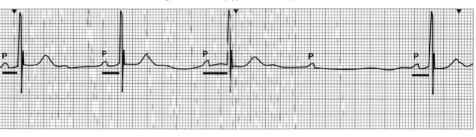

Second-Degree AV Block (Type I AV Block [Wenckebach])

▬▬ = PR interval

P Waves: Those of the underlying rhythm; periodically a QRS complex fails to occur after a P wave (nonconducted P wave or dropped beat).

PR Intervals: Gradually lengthen until a dropped beat occurs, after which the sequence begins anew.

R-R Intervals: Unequal; gradually decrease as the PR intervals lengthen until a dropped beat occurs, resulting in a prolonged R-R interval. Following this, the cycle begins anew.

QRS Complexes: Usually normal (0.12 second or less), unless a preexisting intraventricular conduction delay is present.

AV Conduction Ratio: Commonly, the AV conduction ratio is 5:4, 4:3, or 3:2, but it may be 6:5, 7:6, and so forth.

Treatment: See Section III, page 94.

Second-Degree AV Block, Type II AV Block

Rate: The atrial rate is that of the underlying rhythm. The ventricular rate is typically less than the atrial rate.

Regularity: Patterned irregularity.

P Waves: Those of the underlying rhythm; periodically a QRS complex fails to occur after a P wave (nonconducted P wave or dropped beat).

PR Intervals: May be normal (0.12 to 0.20 second) or abnormal (greater than 0.20 second); usually constant.

R-R Intervals: Unequal.

Second-Degree AV Block (Type II AV Block)

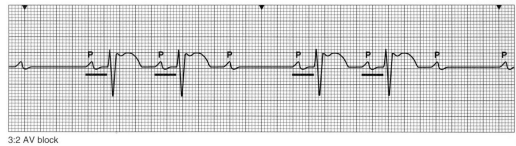

3:2 AV block

━━ = PR interval

QRS Complexes: Usually normal (0.12 second or less), unless a preexisting intraventricular conduction delay is present.

AV Conduction Ratio: The AV conduction ratio is commonly 4:3 or 3:2, but it may be 5:4, 6:5, 7:6, and so forth.

Treatment: See Section III, page 95.

Second-Degree AV Block, 2:1 and Advanced AV Block

Rate: The atrial rate is that of the underlying rhythm. The ventricular rate is typically less than the atrial rate.

Regularity: The atrial rhythm is essentially regular; the ventricular rhythm may be regular or irregular.

2:1 AV block

—— = PR interval

P Waves: Those of the underlying rhythm; periodically, QRS complexes fail to occur after one or more P waves (nonconducted P waves or dropped beats).

PR Intervals: Normal (0.12 to 0.20 second) or abnormal (greater than 0.20 second); usually constant.

R-R Intervals: Equal or may vary.

QRS Complexes: Normal (0.12 second or less) or abnormal (greater than 0.12 second) because of a bundle branch block.

AV Conduction Ratio: Commonly, the AV conduction ratios are even numbers, 2:1, 4:1, 6:1, 8:1, and so forth, but they may be uneven numbers, 3:1 or 5:1. A 3:1 or higher AV block is called an *advanced AV block*.

Treatment: See Section III, page 95.

Third-Degree AV Block

Third-Degree AV Block (Complete AV Block)

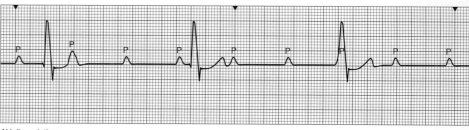

AV dissociation

Rate: The atrial rate is typically 60 to 100 beats/min. The ventricular rate is typically 40 to 60 beats/min (but may be 30 to 40 beats/min or less) and independent of the atrial rate (AV dissociation).

Regularity: The atrial rhythm is that of the underlying rhythm: regular or irregular. The ventricular rhythm is essentially regular.

P Waves: The P waves occur independently of the QRS complexes.

PR Intervals: None.

R-R Intervals: Usually equal.

QRS Complexes: Usually abnormal (greater than 0.12 second).

Site of Origin: The pacemaker site of the P waves is the SA node or an ectopic pacemaker in the atria or AV junction. The pacemaker site of the QRS complexes is an escape pacemaker in the AV junction (junctional escape rhythm) or ventricles (ventricular escape rhythm).

Treatment: See Section III, page 95.

3

Dysrhythmia Management

Paroxysmal Supraventricular Tachycardia (PSVT) with Narrow QRS Complexes (without Wolff-Parkinson-White Syndrome or Ventricular Preexcitation)

Junctional Tachycardia

Atrial Flutter/Atrial Fibrillation (Without Wolff-Parkinson-White Syndrome or Ventricular Preexcitation)

Atrial Flutter/Atrial Fibrillation (with Wolff-Parkinson-White Syndrome or Ventricular Preexcitation)

Wide QRS Complex Tachycardia of Unknown Origin (with Pulse)

Ventricular Tachycardia (VT), Monomorphic (with Pulse)

Ventricular Tachycardia (VT), Polymorphic (with Pulse) Normal Baseline QT Interval

Ventricular Tachycardia (VT), Polymorphic (with Pulse) Prolonged Baseline QT Interval

Torsades de Pointes (TdP) (with Pulse)

Premature Atrial Complexes (PACS)

Premature Junctional Complexes (PJCS)

Premature Ventricular Complexes (PVCS)

Ventricular Fibrillation (VF)

Pulseless Ventricular Tachycardia (VT)

Asystole

Pulseless Electrical Activity

Pharmacological Therapy

Procainamide End Point
- Tachycardia is suppressed.
- A total dose of 17 mg/kg of procainamide has been administered (1.2 g of procainamide for a 70-kg patient).
- Side effects from the procainamide appear (such as hypotension).
- The QRS complex widens by 50% of its original width.

Administration of Calcium Channel Blockers: Calcium channel blockers are contraindicated in the following circumstances:
- If hypotension or cardiogenic shock is present
- If second- or third-degree atrioventricular (AV) block, sinus node dysfunction, atrial flutter or fibrillation associated with ventricular or atrio-His preexcitation, or a wide QRS complex tachycardia is present
- If β-blockers are being administered intravenously (IV)
- If there is a history of bradycardia

Use calcium channel blockers cautiously, if at all, in patients with congestive heart failure and in those receiving oral β-blockers.

Monitor the patient's blood pressure and pulse frequently during and after the administration of a calcium channel blocker.

If hypotension occurs with a calcium channel blocker, place the patient in a Trendelenburg position and administer 1 g of calcium chloride IV slowly, intravenous fluids, and a vasopressor.

If bradycardia, AV block, or asystole occurs, refer to the appropriate treatment protocol.

Administration of β-Blockers: β-Blockers are contraindicated in the following circumstances:
- If bradycardia (heart rate <60 beats/min) is present
- If hypotension (systolic blood pressure <100 mm Hg) is present
- If PR interval is greater than 0.24 second or second- or third-degree AV block is present
- If severe congestive heart failure (left- and/or right-sided heart failure) is present
- If bronchospasm or a history of asthma is present (relative contraindication)
- If severe chronic obstructive pulmonary disease (COPD) is present
- If intravenous calcium channel blockers have been administered within a few hours (caution advised)

Monitor the patient's blood pressure and pulse frequently during and after the administration of a β-blocker.

If hypotension occurs with a β-blocker, place the patient in a Trendelenburg position and administer a vasopressor.

If bradycardia, AV block, or asystole occurs, refer to the appropriate treatment protocol.

Cardioversion and Defibrillation

Defibrillation

Pulseless ventricular tachycardia (VT)/ventricular fibrillation (VF)	360 J monophasic, 120-200 J biphasic
Sustained polymorphic VT	360 J monophasic, 120-200 J biphasic

Synchronized cardioversion

Narrow complex-QRS tachycardia	50 J, 100 J, 100 J, 200 J, 300 J, 360 J*
Atrial flutter with rapid ventricular response (RVR)	50 J, 100 J, 100 J, 200 J, 300 J, 360 J*
Atrial fibrillation with RVR	100-120 J, 200 J, 300 J, 360 J*
VT with a pulse	100-120 J, 200 J, 300 J, 360 J*

---

* Or biphasic equivalent.

Sedation: When performing cardioversion, remember that this procedure will cause the patient pain and anxiety, and therefore vascular access will be required to administer analgesics and sedatives. In addition, the patient will usually require higher doses than are used for transcutaneous pacing. The following are agents to consider for sedation:

- Administer 2 to 4 mg of **midazolam** IV slowly, repeat every 3 to 5 minutes, titrate to produce sedation/amnesia.

OR

- Administer 5 to 10 mg **diazepam** IV, repeat every 3 to 5 minutes, titrate to produce sedation/amnesia.

OR

- Administer 6 mg **etomidate** IV (0.2 to 0.6 mg/kg), repeat every 3 to 5 minutes, titrate to produce sedation/amnesia.

If the patient is in pain, consider the following agents in addition to any of the previous agents:

- Administer 2 to 5 mg **morphine** IV slowly to produce analgesia.

OR

- Administer 1 μg/kg **fentanyl** IV to produce analgesia; may repeat 0.5 μg/kg **fentanyl** if sufficient analgesia is not produced within 5 to 10 minutes.

Transcutaneous Pacing

Transcutaneous pacing (TCP) is usually effective in the treatment of all symptomatic bradycardias, regardless of cause.

The indications for TCP are as follows:

- TCP is indicated in the treatment of all symptomatic bradycardias resistant to pharmacologic therapy.
- TCP is indicated in the initial treatment of the following symptomatic bradycardias with wide QRS complexes when vascular access is delayed or dysrhythmia is resistant to pharmacologic therapy:
  - Second-degree, type II AV block
  - Second-degree, 2:1 and advanced AV block with wide QRS complexes
  - Third-degree AV block with wide QRS complexes
- TCP should be considered in the initial treatment of symptomatic bradycardias associated with acute coronary syndromes in situations in which vascular access is difficult or delayed.
- TCP is the treatment of choice in symptomatic bradycardias in patients with heart transplants because atropine sulfate is usually ineffective in such patients.

Contraindications for TCP follow:

- TCP is not indicated in bradycardia caused by hypothermia.

It is reasonable to attempt a trial of a pharmacological agent to treat the bradycardia while preparing the transcutaneous pacemaker.

Sinus Bradycardia

Sinus Arrest/Sinoatrial (SA) Exit Block

Second-Degree, Type I AV Block (Wenckebach)

Second-Degree, 2:1 and Advanced AV Block with Narrow QRS Complexes

Third-Degree AV Block with Narrow QRS Complexes

A bradycardia is considered "symptomatic" when one or more of the following clinical conditions or signs or symptoms are present:

- Hypotension or shock (systolic blood pressure <90 mm Hg)
- Congestive heart failure, pulmonary congestion
- Chest pain or dyspnea
- Decreased level of consciousness caused by decreased cardiac output
- Premature ventricular complexes (PVCs), particularly in the setting of an acute MI

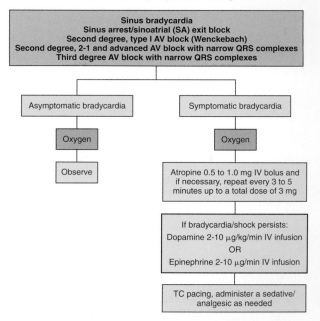

Sinus bradycardia
Sinus arrest/sinoatrial (SA) exit block
Second degree, type I AV block (Wenckebach)
Second degree, 2-1 and advanced AV block with narrow QRS complexes
Third degree AV block with narrow QRS complexes

Asymptomatic bradycardia

Oxygen

Observe

Symptomatic bradycardia

Oxygen

Atropine 0.5 to 1.0 mg IV bolus and if necessary, repeat every 3 to 5 minutes up to a total dose of 3 mg

If bradycardia/shock persists:
Dopamine 2-10 μg/kg/min IV infusion
OR
Epinephrine 2-10 μg/min IV infusion

TC pacing, administer a sedative/analgesic as needed

Second-Degree, Type II AV Block

Second-Degree, 2:1 and Advanced
AV Block with Wide QRS Complexes

Third-Degree AV Block with Wide
QRS Complexes

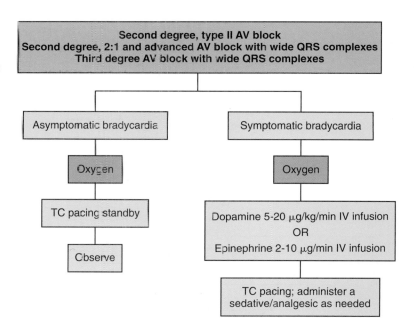

Junctional Escape Rhythm

Ventricular Escape Rhythm

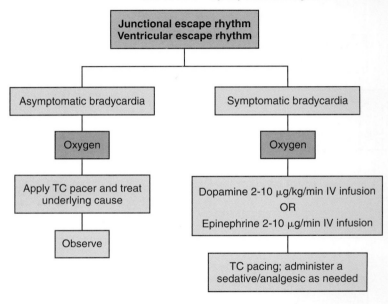

Sinus Tachycardia

Patient's condition stable or unstable

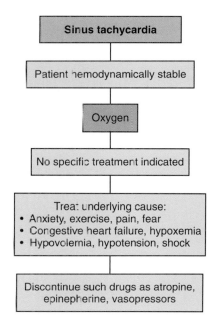

Atrial Tachycardia without Block

A patient's condition is considered "unstable" when one or more of the following clinical conditions or signs or symptoms are present:

- Hypotension or shock (systolic blood pressure 90 mm Hg or less)
- Congestive heart failure, pulmonary congestion
- Chest pain or dyspnea
- Decreased level of consciousness caused by decreased cardiac output
- Acute MI

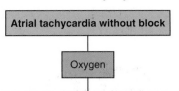

Atrial tachycardia without block

Oxygen

Diltiazem 20 mg (0.25 mg/kg) IV bolus over 2 minutes and, if necessary, in 15 minutes administer a 25 mg (0.35 mg/kg) IV bolus over 2 minutes followed by an IV infusion at a rate of 5 to 15 mg/hr

OR

One of the following beta blockers:

Esmolol 0.5 mg/kg IV bolus over 1 minute followed by an IV infusion at a rate of 0.05 mg/kg/min; repeat the IV bolus twice, 5 minutes between each bolus, while increasing the rate of the IV infusion 0.05 mg/kg/min every 5 minutes to a maximum of 0.20 mg/kg/min

Atenolol 2.5 - 5 mg IV over 5 minutes and repeat in 10 minutes for a total dose of 10 mg

Metoprolol 5 mg IV over 2 to 3 minutes and repeat every 5 minutes up to a total dose of 15 mg

OR

Amiodarone 150 mg IV infusion over 10 minutes followed by a 1 mg/min IV infusion

Atrial Tachycardia with Block

Patient's condition stable or unstable.

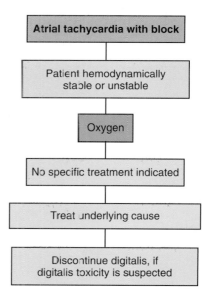

Atrial tachycardia with block

Patient hemodynamically stable or unstable

Oxygen

No specific treatment indicated

Treat underlying cause

Discontinue digitalis, if digitalis toxicity is suspected

Narrow QRS Complex Tachycardia of Unknown Origin (with Pulse)

If the dysrhythmia converts to a sinus rhythm at any time, indicating that paroxysmal supraventricular tachycardia (PSVT) is present, continue with the appropriate step in the section on *Paroxysmal Supraventricular Tachycardia with Narrow QRS Complexes*, page 101.

If the heart rate slows at any time, indicating that an atrial tachycardia is present, continue with the treatment plans outlined in either the section on *Atrial Tachycardia Without Block* (subsequent) or the section on *Junctional Tachycardia* (page 102), as appropriate.

If the heart rate slows at any time, indicating an underlying atrial fibrillation or atrial flutter rhythm, continue with the treatment plans outlined in the section on *Atrial Flutter/Atrial Fibrillation* (pages 103-105) as appropriate.

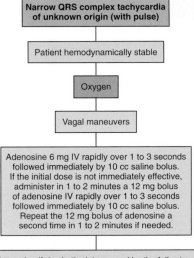

Paroxysmal
Supraventricular
Tachycardia (PSVT)
with Narrow QRS
Complexes
(without Wolff-
Parkinson-White
Syndrome or
Ventricular
Preexcitation)

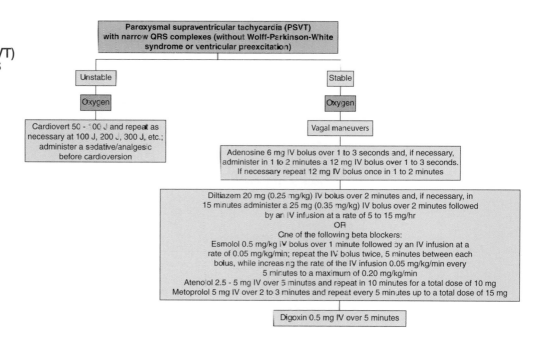

Junctional Tachycardia

Monitor the pulse, blood pressure, and ECG while
administering the drug. Stop the administration of
the β-blocker if the systolic blood pressure falls below
100 mm Hg.

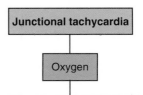

Junctional tachycardia

Oxygen

Amiodarone 150 mg IV infusion over 10 minutes
followed by a 1 mg/min IV infusion

OR

One of the following beta blockers:

Esmolol 0.5 mg/kg IV bolus over 1 minute followed by an IV infusion at a
rate of 0.05 mg/kg/min; repeat the IV bolus twice, 5 minutes between each
bolus, while increasing the rate of the IV infusion 0.05 mg/kg/min after
each bolus. Then if necessary, increase the IV infusion by .0.5 mg/kg/min
every 5 minutes to a maximum of 0.20 mg/kg/min

Atenolol 2.5 - 5 mg IV over 5 minutes and repeat in 10 minutes
for a total dose of 10 mg

Metoprolol 5 mg IV over 2 to 3 minutes and repeat
every 5 minutes up to a total dose of 15 mg

Atrial Flutter/Atrial Fibrillation (without Wolff-Parkinson-White Syndrome or Ventricular Preexcitation)

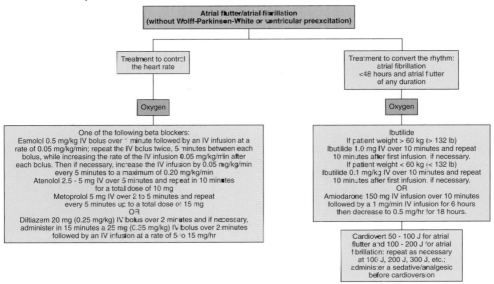

Atrial flutter/atrial fibrillation
(without Wolff-Parkinson-White or ventricular preexcitation)

Treatment to control the heart rate

Oxygen

One of the following beta blockers:
Esmolol 0.5 mg/kg IV bolus over 1 minute followed by an IV infusion at a rate of 0.05 mg/kg/min; repeat the IV bolus twice, 5 minutes between each bolus, while increasing the rate of the IV infusion 0.05 mg/kg/min after each bolus. Then if necessary, increase the IV infusion by 0.05 mg/kg/min every 5 minutes to a maximum of 0.20 mg/kg/min
Atenolol 2.5 - 5 mg IV over 5 minutes and repeat in 10 minutes for a total dose of 10 mg
Metoprolol 5 mg IV over 2 to 5 minutes and repeat every 5 minutes up to a total dose of 15 mg
OR
Diltiazem 20 mg (0.25 mg/kg) IV bolus over 2 minutes and if necessary, administer in 15 minutes a 25 mg (0.35 mg/kg) IV bolus over 2 minutes followed by an IV infusion at a rate of 5 to 15 mg/hr

---

Treatment to convert the rhythm:
atrial fibrillation <48 hours and atrial flutter of any duration

Oxygen

Ibutilide
If patient weight > 60 kg (> 132 lb)
Ibutilide 1.0 mg IV over 10 minutes and repeat 10 minutes after first infusion. if necessary.
If patient weight < 60 kg (< 132 lb)
Ibutilide 0.1 mg/kg IV over 10 minutes and repeat 10 minutes after first infusion. if necessary.
OR
Amiodarone 150 mg IV infusion over 10 minutes followed by a 1 mg/min IV infusion for 6 hours then decrease to 0.5 mg/hr for 18 hours.

Cardiovert 50 - 100 J for atrial flutter and 100 - 200 J for atrial fibrillation: repeat as necessary at 100 J, 200 J, 300 J, etc.; administer a sedative/analgesic before cardioversion

Atrial Fibrillation >48 Hours or of Unknown Duration

Rhythm conversion is contraindicated until the patient has been anticoagulated with heparin. There is an increased risk of a thromboembolic event resulting in stroke because of thrombus formation that may have occurred during the period of atrial fibrillation.

If patient becomes unstable or amiodarone fails to convert rhythm, perform immediate synchronized cardioversion.

For Atrial Fibrillation: Cardiovert at 100-200 J with a monophasic waveform.
Cardiovert at 100-120 J with a biphasic waveform.
Escalate subsequent shock doses as required.

For Atrial Flutter: Cardiovert at 50-100 J with a monophasic waveform.
Escalate subsequent shock doses as required.
AND

Administer an antiarrhythmic drug such as **amiodarone** (if not already administered).

Administer a loading dose of 150 mg of amiodarone IV over 10 minutes.
AND

Start an intravenous infusion of amiodarone at a rate of 1 mg/min for 6 hours then decrease to 0.5 mg/min for 18 hours.

Atrial Flutter/Atrial Fibrillation (with Wolff-Parkinson-White Syndrome or Ventricular Preexcitation)

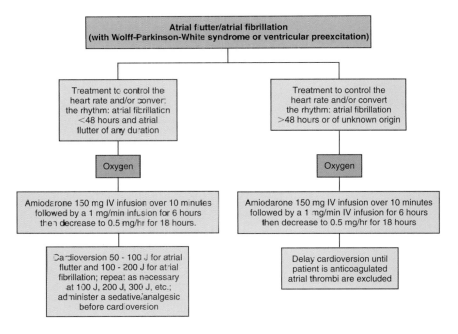

Atrial flutter/atrial fibrillation
(with Wolff-Parkinson-White syndrome or ventricular preexcitation)

(Left branch)

Treatment to control the heart rate and/or convert the rhythm: atrial fibrillation <48 hours and atrial flutter of any duration

Oxygen

Amiodarone 150 mg IV infusion over 10 minutes followed by a 1 mg/min infusion for 6 hours then decrease to 0.5 mg/hr for 18 hours.

Cardioversion 50 - 100 J for atrial flutter and 100 - 200 J for atrial fibrillation; repeat as necessary at 100 J, 200 J, 300 J, etc.; administer a sedative/analgesic before cardioversion

(Right branch)

Treatment to control the heart rate and/or convert the rhythm: atrial fibrillation >48 hours or of unknown origin

Oxygen

Amiodarone 150 mg IV infusion over 10 minutes followed by a 1 mg/min IV infusion for 6 hours then decrease to 0.5 mg/hr for 18 hours

Delay cardioversion until patient is anticoagulated atrial thrombi are excluded

Wide QRS Complex Tachycardia of Unknown Origin (with Pulse)

If the wide QRS complex tachycardia persists and the patient becomes pulseless at any time:

- Continue with *Ventricular Fibrillation/ Pulseless Ventricular Tachycardia,* page 113.

If electrical or pharmacological therapy is successful in terminating the wide QRS complex tachycardia:

- Continue or start a maintenance intravenous infusion of amiodarone or procainamide as appropriate.

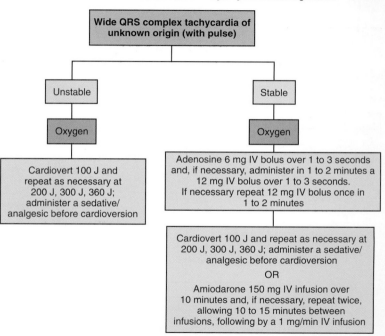

Wide QRS complex tachycardia of unknown origin (with pulse)

Unstable

Oxygen

Cardiovert 100 J and repeat as necessary at 200 J, 300 J, 360 J; administer a sedative/ analgesic before cardioversion

Stable

Oxygen

Adenosine 6 mg IV bolus over 1 to 3 seconds and, if necessary, administer in 1 to 2 minutes a 12 mg IV bolus over 1 to 3 seconds. If necessary repeat 12 mg IV bolus once in 1 to 2 minutes

Cardiovert 100 J and repeat as necessary at 200 J, 300 J, 360 J; administer a sedative/ analgesic before cardioversion

OR

Amiodarone 150 mg IV infusion over 10 minutes and, if necessary, repeat twice, allowing 10 to 15 minutes between infusions, following by a 1 mg/min IV infusion

Ventricular Tachycardia (VT), Monomorphic (with Pulse)

If one of the shocks or medications is successful in terminating ventricular tachycardia:

- Continue or start a maintenance intravenous infusion of amiodarone, lidocaine, or procainamide as appropriate.

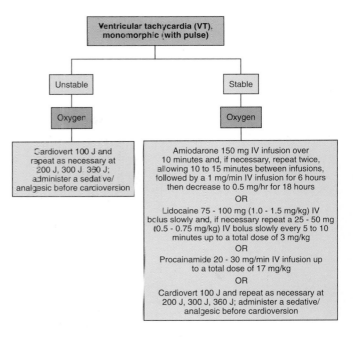

Ventricular Tachycardia (VT),
Polymorphic (with Pulse) Normal
Baseline QT Interval

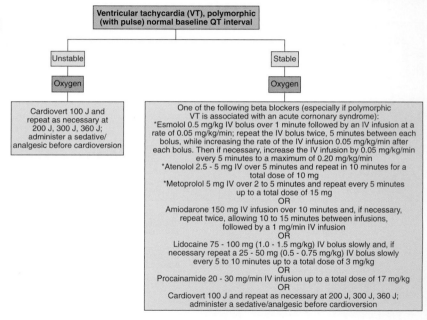

If a β-blocker, amiodarone, lidocaine, or procainamide is unsuccessful in suppressing the polymorphic ventricular tachycardia, or if at any time while administering the β-blocker, procainamide, amiodarone, or lidocaine, the patient's condition becomes hemodynamically unstable and cardioversions were not delivered initially:

- Immediately deliver a cardioversion (200 J), premedicating the patient first if necessary

AND

- Repeat the cardioversion as often as necessary at progressively increasing energy levels (200 to 300 J and 360 J).

If one of the shocks or medications is successful in terminating the polymorphic ventricular tachycardia:

- Continue or start a maintenance intravenous infusion of the β-blocker, amiodarone, lidocaine, or procainamide as appropriate.

**Ventricular
Tachycardia (VT),
Polymorphic
(with Pulse)**

**Prolonged
Baseline QT
Interval**

**Torsades de
Pointes (TdP)
(with Pulse)**

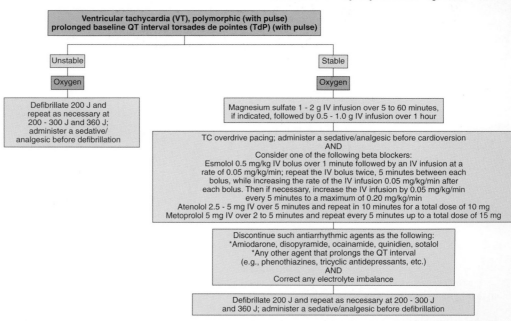

If polymorphic ventricular tachycardia or torsades de pointes degenerates into ventricular fibrillation at any time:

- Continue with *Ventricular Fibrillation/Pulseless Ventricular Tachycardia,* page 113.

Premature Atrial Complexes (PACs)

Premature Junctional Complexes (PJCs)

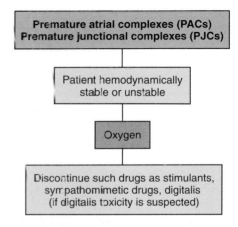

Premature Ventricular Complexes (PVCs)

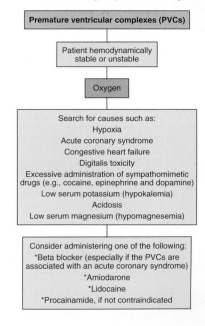

Premature ventricular complexes (PVCs)

Patient hemodynamically stable or unstable

Oxygen

Search for causes such as:
Hypoxia
Acute coronary syndrome
Congestive heart failure
Digitalis toxicity
Excessive administration of sympathomimetic drugs (e.g., cocaine, epinephrine and dopamine)
Low serum potassium (hypokalemia)
Acidosis
Low serum magnesium (hypomagnesemia)

Consider administering one of the following:
*Beta blocker (especially if the PVCs are associated with an acute coronary syndrome)
*Amiodarone
*Lidocaine
*Procainamide, if not contraindicated

Ventricular Fibrillation (VF)

Pulseless Ventricular Tachycardia (VT)

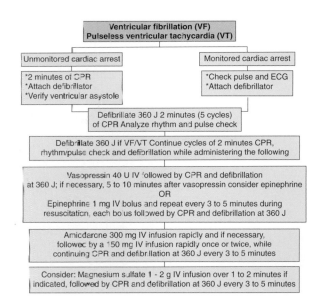

Asystole

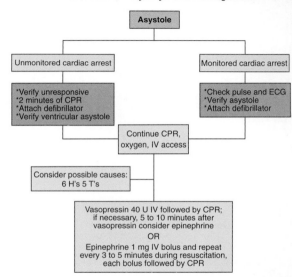

Pulseless Electrical Activity
6 Hs and 5 Ts

- Hypovolemia: administer 250- to 500-mL bolus of **normal saline,** repeat as needed
- Hypoxia: ensure adequate oxygenation
- Hydrogen ion/Acidosis: ensure adequate ventilation
- Hyperkalemia/Hypokalemia: correct with appropriate electrolyte
- Hypoglycemia
- Hypothermia: rewarm
- Toxins/Drug overdose: administer antidote
- Tamponade—cardiac: perform pericardiocentesis
- Tension pneumothorax: perform needle decompression
- Thrombosis: identify myocardial infarction or pulmonary embolism
- Trauma

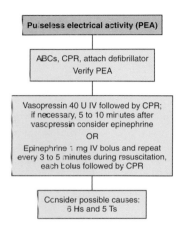

Pulseless electrical activity (PEA)

ABCs, CPR, attach defibrillator
Verify PEA

Vasopressin 40 U IV followed by CPR;
if necessary, 5 to 10 minutes after
vasopressin consider epinephrine
OR
Epinephrine 1 mg IV bolus and repeat
every 3 to 5 minutes during resuscitation,
each bolus followed by CPR

Consider possible causes:
6 Hs and 5 Ts

Postresuscitation Management

In the event that return of spontaneous circulation (ROSC) occurs, the initial objectives of postresuscitation care are to do the following:

- Optimize cardiopulmonary function and systemic perfusion, especially perfusion to the brain.
- Transport the victim of out-of-hospital cardiac arrest or hospital emergency department (ED) to an appropriately equipped critical care unit.
- Try to identify the precipitating causes of the arrest.
- Institute measures to prevent recurrence.
- Institute measures that may improve long-term, neurologically intact survival.

Airway

- Ensure airway is properly secured and patient is easy to ventilate.
- Assess pulse oximetry continuously.
- Maintain end-tidal CO_2 between 35 and 45 mm Hg. If less than 35 mm Hg, slow ventilation rate. If greater than 45 mm Hg, increase ventilation rate.

Circulation

- Assess presence of pulses and attempt to obtain blood pressure.
- If hypotension and *signs and symptoms of shock are present:*
  - Systolic blood pressure less than 70 mm Hg:
    Start an intravenous infusion of norepinephrine at an initial rate of 0.5 to 1 μg/min, and adjust the rate of infusion up to 8 to 30 μg/min to increase the systolic blood pressure to 70 to 100 mm Hg.
    OR
  - Systolic blood pressure 70 to 100 mm Hg:
    Start an intravenous infusion of **dopamine** at an initial rate of 2 to 10 μg/kg/min, and adjust the rate of infusion up to 20 μg/kg/min to increase the systolic blood pressure to 90 to 100 mm Hg or greater.
- If hypertensive, monitor frequently.

Neurologic

- Assess level of consciousness.
- Sedate patient if combative and in danger of dislodging airway.

Metabolic

- Obtain blood glucose and administer **D50** if less than 70 mg/dL; administer **insulin** if greater than 200 mg/dL.

Temperature Control

- Do not attempt to warm patient unless severe hypothermia is the suspected cause of the arrest.
- Consider induced hypothermia if hospital is equipped to perform.

Rate and Rhythm Control

- If a symptomatic post-defibrillation dysrhythmia is present:
  - Refer to the appropriate algorithm for treatment.
- If rhythm was converted with the administration of an antidysrhythmic, consider continuation of an infusion of that agent.

Consider prophylactic administration of an antidysrhythmic agent.

Bundle Branch and Fascicular Blocks

4

Right Bundle Branch Block (RBBB)
Left Bundle Branch Block (LBBB)
Left Anterior Fascicular Block (LAFB)

Left Posterior Fascicular Block (LPFB)
Bifascicular Blocks—RBBB with LAFB
Bifascicular Blocks—RBBB with LPFB

Right Bundle Branch Block (RBBB)

QRS Duration: Greater than 0.12 second in complete RBBB; 0.10 to 0.12 second in incomplete RBBB.

QRS Axis: Normal or slight right axis deviation (+90° to +110°).

ST Segments: May be depressed in leads V_1-V_3.

T Waves: May be inverted in leads V_1-V_3.

QRS Complexes: With an intact interventricular septum(no previous septal myocardial infarction)
- Leads V_1 and V_2
  - Wide QRS with a classic triphasic rSR′ ("M" or "rabbit ears") pattern:
    - Initial small r wave
    - Deep, slurred S wave
    - Terminal tall R′ wave

- Leads I, aVL, and V_5-V_6
  - Wide QRS with a typical qRS pattern:
    - Initial small q wave
    - Tall R wave
    - Terminal deep, slurred S wave

QRS Complexes: Without an intact interventricular septum (previous septal myocardial infarction)
- Leads V_1 and V_2
  - Wide QRS with a QSR pattern:
    - Absent initial small r wave
    - Deep QS wave
    - Terminal tall R wave
- Leads I, aVL, and V_5-V_6
  - Wide QRS with an RS pattern:
    - Absent initial small q wave
    - Tall R wave
    - Terminal deep, slurred S wave

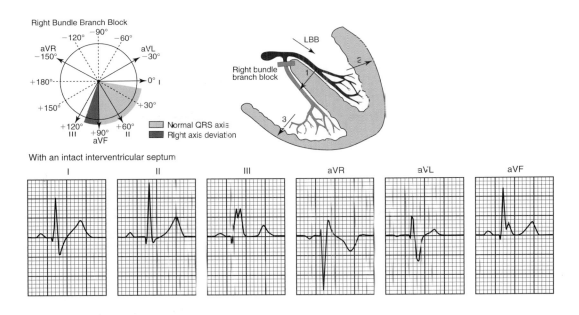

Right Bundle Branch Block

Normal QRS axis
Right axis deviation

LBB

Right bundle branch block

With an intact interventricular septum

I   II   III   aVR   aVL   aVF

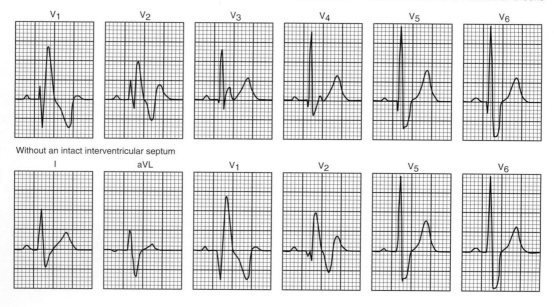

Without an intact interventricular septum

Left Bundle Branch Block (LBBB)

QRS Duration: Greater than 0.12 second in complete LBBB; 0.10 to 0.12 second in incomplete LBBB.

QRS Axis: Commonly, left axis deviation ($-30°$ to $-90°$), but may be normal.

ST Segments: Depressed in leads I, aVL, and V_5-V_6; elevated in leads V_1-V_3.

T Waves: Inverted in leads I, aVL, and V_5-V_6; elevated in leads V_1-V_3.

QRS Complexes: With an intact interventricular septum (no previous septal myocardial infarction)

- Leads V_1-V_3
  - Wide QRS with an rS or QS pattern:
    - Initial small r wave
    - Deep, wide S wave
      OR
    - Absent R wave
    - Deep, wide QS wave
- Leads I, aVL, and V_5-V_6
  - Wide QRS with an R pattern:
    - Absent initial small q wave
    - Tall, wide, slurred R wave with or without notching, and a prolonged ventricular activation time (VAT)

Without an intact interventricular septum (previous septal myocardial infarction)

- Leads V_1 and V_2
  - Wide QRS with an rS pattern:
    - Small, narrow r wave
    - Deep, wide S wave
- Leads I, aVL, and V_5-V_6
  - Wide QRS with a qR pattern:
    - Small q wave
    - Tall, wide, slurred R wave with or without notching, and a prolonged VAT

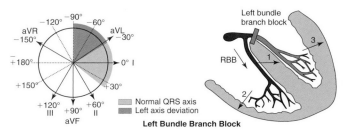

Normal QRS axis

Left axis deviation

Left Bundle Branch Block

With an intact interventricular septum

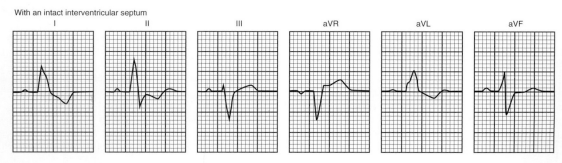

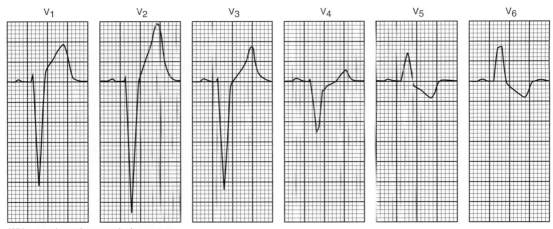

Without an intact interventricular septum

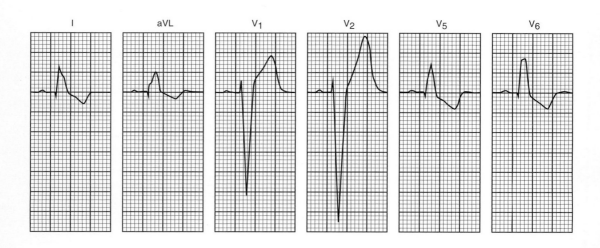

Left Anterior Fascicular Block (LAFB)

QRS Duration: Normal, less than 0.12 second.

QRS Axis: Left axis deviation (−30° to −90°).

ST Segments: Normal.

T Waves: Normal.

QRS Complexes:
- Leads I and aVL
    - Narrow QRS
        - Initial small q wave
- Leads II, III, and aVF
    - Narrow QRS
        - Initial small r wave
        - Deep S wave, typically larger than the R wave

QRS Pattern: A typical q_1r_3 pattern is present.

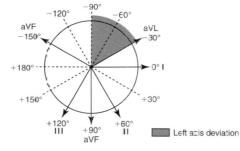

Left Anterior Fascicular Block

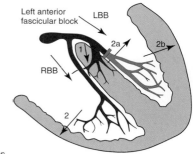

I	II	III	aVR	aVL	aVF

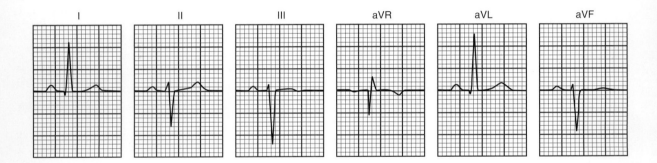

Left Posterior Fascicular Block (LPFB)

QRS Duration: Normal, less than 0.12 second.

QRS Axis: Right axis deviation (+110° to +180°).

ST Segments: Normal.

T Waves: Normal.

QRS Complexes:

- Leads I, aVL, and V_5-V_6
  - Narrow QRS
    - Absent q wave in leads I, aVL, and V_5-V_6
    - Initial small r wave in leads I and aVL
    - Deep S wave in leads I and aVL
- Leads II, III, and aVF
  - Narrow QRS
    - Initial small q wave
    - Tall R wave

QRS Pattern: A typical q_3r_1 pattern is present.

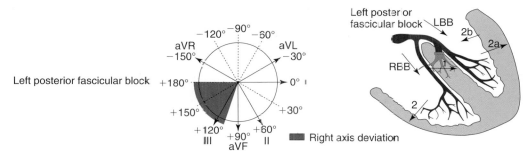

Left posterior fascicular block

Right axis deviation

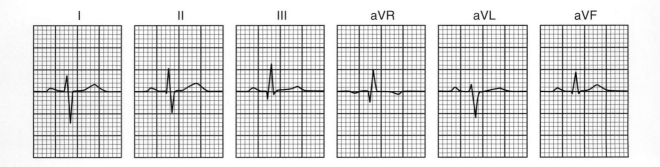

Bifascicular Blocks—
RBBB with LAFB

QRS Duration: Greater than 0.12 second.

QRS Axis: Left axis deviation (−30° to −90°).

ST Segments: Normal.

T Waves: Normal.

QRS Complexes:
- Typical RBBB with RSR′ in V_1 and slurred S in V_6
- rS pattern in III typical of LAFB

Bifascicular block right bundle branch block with left anterior fascicular block

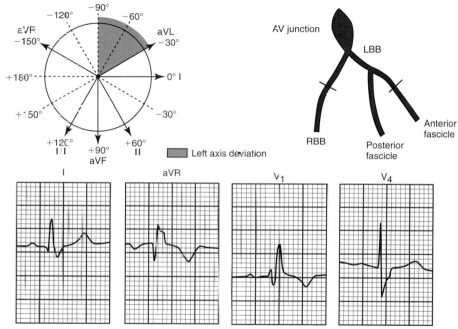

Left axis deviation

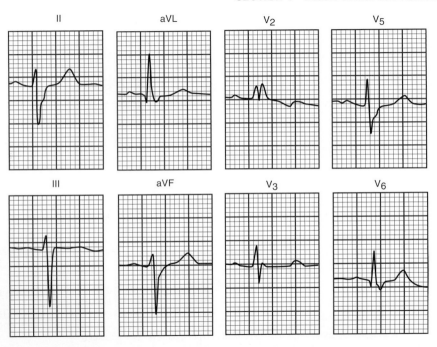

II	aVL	V₂	V₅
III	aVF	V₃	V₆

Bifascicular Blocks— RBBB with LPFB

QRS Duration: Greater than 0.12 second.

QRS Axis: Right axis deviation (+110° to +180°).

ST Segments: Normal.

T Waves: Normal.

QRS Complexes:

- Typical configuration of RBBB with RSR′ pattern in V_1 and slurred S in V_6
- Small q wave in III typical of LAFB

Bifascicular block: right bundle branch block with left posterior fascicular block

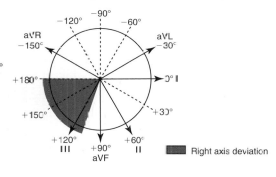

Right axis deviation

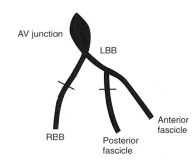

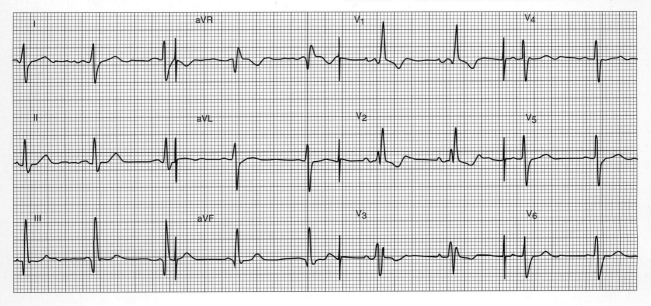

5

Other Assorted ECG Changes

Chamber Enlargement
Right Atrial Enlargement
Left Atrial Enlargement
Right Ventricular Hypertrophy (RVH)
Left Ventricular Hypertrophy (LVH)
Pericarditis
Electrolyte Imbalance
Hyperkalemia
Hypokalemia
Hypercalcemia
Hypocalcemia
Drug Effect
Digitalis

Procainamide
Pulmonary Disease
Pulmonary Embolism (Acute)
Chronic Cor Pulmonale
Early Repolarization
Hypothermia
Preexcitation Syndromes
Ventricular Preexcitation
Atrio-His Preexcitation
Nodoventricular/Fasciculoventricular Preexcitation
Brugada syndrome

CHAMBER ENLARGEMENT

Right Atrial Enlargement

P Waves:

Duration: Usually normal (0.10 second or less).

Shape: Typically tall and symmetrically peaked P waves in leads II, III, and aVF—the P pulmonale. Sharply peaked biphasic P waves in lead V_1-V_2.

Direction: Positive (upright) in leads II, III, and aVF; biphasic in V_1-V_2, with the initial deflection greater than the terminal deflection.

Amplitude: 2.5 mm or greater in leads II, III, and aVF.

Cause of Right Atrial Enlargement (Right Atrial Dilatation and Hypertrophy): Increased pressure and/or volume in the right atrium (i.e., right atrial overload), commonly the result of the following:

- Pulmonary valve stenosis
- Tricuspid valve stenosis and insufficiency (relatively rare)
- Pulmonary hypertension from various causes, including chronic obstructive pulmonary disease (COPD), status asthmaticus, pulmonary embolism, pulmonary edema, mitral valve stenosis or insufficiency, and congenital heart disease

The result of right atrial enlargement is typically a tall, symmetrically peaked P wave—the **P pulmonale.**

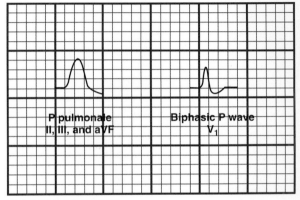

Right atrial enlargement

Left Atrial Enlargement

P Waves:

Duration: Usually greater than 0.10 second.

Shape:

- A broad positive (upright) P wave, 0.10 second or greater in duration, in any lead.
- A wide, notched P wave with two "humps" 0.04 second or more apart—the *P mitrale,* usually present in leads I, II, and V₄-V₆. The first hump represents the depolarization of the right atrium; the second hump represents the depolarization of the enlarged left atrium.
- A biphasic P wave, greater than 0.10 second in total duration, with the terminal, negative component 1 mm (0.10 mV) or more deep and 1 mm (0.04 second) or more in duration (i.e., 1 small square or greater), commonly present in leads V₁-V₂. The initial, positive (upright) component of the P wave represents the depolarization of the right atrium; the terminal, negative component represents the depolarization of the enlarged left atrium.

Direction: Positive (upright) in leads I, II, and V₄-V₆ and biphasic in leads V₁-V₂; may be negative in leads III and aVF.

Amplitude: Usually normal (0.5 to 2.5 mm).

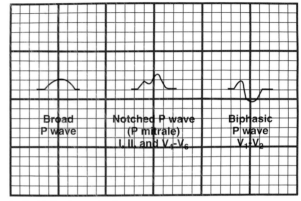

Left atrial enlargement

Cause of Left Atrial Enlargement (Left Atrial Dilatation and Hypertrophy): Increased pressure and/or volume in the left atrium (i.e., left atrial overload), commonly the result of the following:

- Mitral valve stenosis and insufficiency
- Acute myocardial infarction (MI)
- Left-sided heart failure
- Left ventricular hypertrophy from various causes, such as aortic stenosis or insufficiency, systemic hypertension, and hypertrophic cardiomyopathy

The result of left atrial enlargement is typically a wide, notched P wave—the **P mitrale.** Such P waves may also result from a delay or block of the progression of the electrical impulses through the interatrial conduction tract between the right and left atria.

Right Ventricular Hypertrophy (RVH)

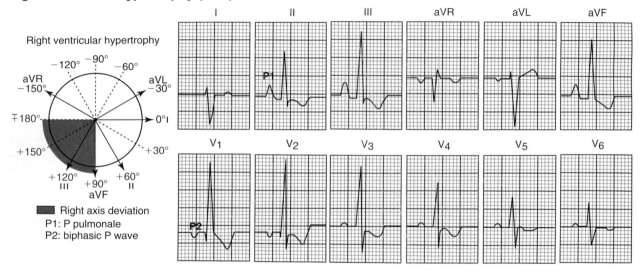

Right ventricular hypertrophy

Right axis deviation
P1: P pulmonale
P2: biphasic P wave

P Waves: Right atrial enlargement usually present.

QRS Complexes
Duration: Normal, 0.12 second or less.
Ventricular Activation Time (VAT): Prolonged beyond the upper normal limit of 0.035 second in leads V_1-V_2.
Q Waves: May be present in leads II, III, and aVF.
R Waves: Tall R waves in leads II, III, and V_1. Usually 7 mm or more (>0.7 mV) in height and equal to or greater than the S waves in depth in lead V_1. Relatively tall R waves also in leads V_2-V_3.
Note: Tall R waves equal to or greater than the S waves in lead V_1 may also be present in acute posterior MI and in dextrocardia.
S Waves: Relatively deeper than normal in leads I and V_4-V_6. In lead V_6, the depth of the S waves may be greater than the height of the R waves.

ST Segments: "Downsloping" ST-segment depression of 1 mm or more may be present in leads II, III, aVF, and V_1 and sometimes in leads V_2 and V_3.

T Waves: Often inverted in leads II, III, aVF, and V_1 and sometimes in leads V_2 and V_3.
Note: The downsloping ST-segment depression and the T wave inversion together form the "strain" pattern characteristic of longstanding RVH, giving the so-called "hockey stick" appearance to the QRS-ST-T complex.

QRS Axis: Right axis deviation of +90° or more; >+110° in adults; >+120° in the young.

Cause of RVH: Increased pressure and/or volume in the right ventricle (i.e., right ventricular overload), commonly the result of the following:
- Pulmonary valve stenosis and other congenital heart defects (e.g., atrial and ventricular septal defects)
- Tricuspid valve insufficiency (relatively rare)
- Pulmonary hypertension from various causes, including COPD, status asthmaticus, pulmonary embolism, pulmonary edema, and mitral valve stenosis or insufficiency

Left Ventricular Hypertrophy (LVH)

Left ventricular hypertrophy

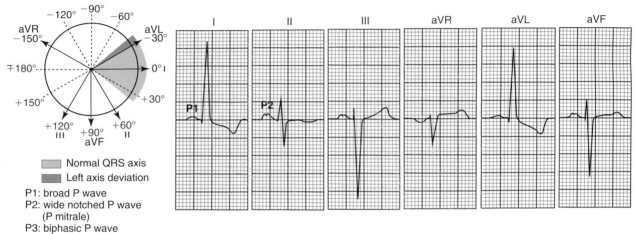

Normal QRS axis

Left axis deviation

P1: broad P wave
P2: wide notched P wave
(P mitrale)
P3: biphasic P wave

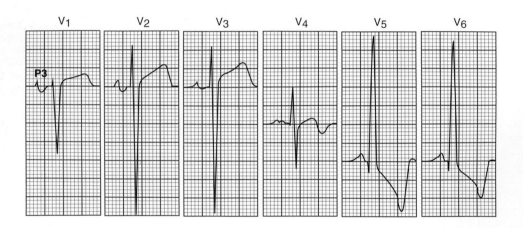

P Waves: Left atrial enlargement usually present.

QRS Complexes
Duration: Normal, 0.12 second or less.
Ventricular Activation Time (VAT): Prolonged beyond the upper normal limit to 0.05 second or more in leads V_5 and V_6.
R Waves: Tall R waves in leads I, aVL, and V_5-V_6.
S Waves: Deep S waves in leads III and V_1-V_2.

QRS Axis: Usually normal, but may be left axis deviation (>−30°).

ST Segments: "Downsloping" ST-segment depression of 1 mm or more in leads I, aVL, and V_5-V_6.

T Waves: Inverted in leads I, aVL, and V_5-V_6. The inverted T waves together with the "downsloping" ST-segment depression form the "strain" pattern characteristic of longstanding LVH—the so-called "hockey stick" appearance of the QRS-ST-T complex.

Diagnosis of LVH: The amplitude (or voltage) of the R waves and the depth (or voltage) of the S waves considered to indicate LVH in certain leads are shown in the following table.

Wave	I	III	aVL	V_1 or V_2	V_5 or V_6
R	>20 mm (>2.0 mV)		>11 mm (>1.1 mV)		>30 mm (>3.0 mV)
S		>20 mm (>2.0 mV)		>30 mm (>3.0 mV)	

Cause of LVH: Increased pressure and/or volume in the left ventricle (i.e., left ventricular overload), commonly the result of the following:

- Mitral insufficiency
- Aortic stenosis or insufficiency
- Systemic hypertension
- Acute MI
- Hypertrophic cardiomyopathy

Sum of R and S Waves: The sum of the amplitude of the R waves and the depth of the S waves (in mm or mV) in certain leads with the most prominent R and S waves is diagnostic of LVH if this sum equals or exceeds the following values:

$$R\,(I, II, \text{ or } III) + S\,(I, II, \text{ or } III) = > 20 \text{ mm } (>2.0 \text{ mV})$$

$$R\,I + S\,III = > 25 \text{ mm } (>2.5 \text{ mV})$$

$$S\,V_1\,(\text{or } S\,V_2) + R\,V_5\,(\text{or } R\,V_6) = > 35 \text{ mm } (>3.5 \text{ mV})$$

Criteria Diagnostic of LVH: LVH is present if criteria 1 and 2 are met:

Criteria 1

$$R\,I \text{ or } S\,III = \geq 20 \text{ mm } (\geq 2.0 \text{ mV})$$

OR

$$R\,I + S\,III = \geq 25 \text{ mm } (\geq 2.5 \text{ mV})$$

OR

$$S\,V_1\,(\text{or } S\,V_2) + R\,V_5\,(\text{or } R\,V_6) = \geq 35 \text{ mm } (\geq 3.5 \text{ mV})$$

Criteria 2

$$\text{QRS axis between } -15° \text{ and } -30° \text{ or greater than } -30°$$
$$(\text{left axis deviation})$$

OR

ST-segment depression of ≥1 mm in leads with an R wave with the amplitude (or voltage) criteria of LVH (see table, p. 143).

Pericarditis

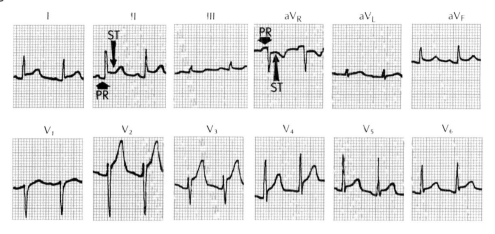

From Goldberger AL: *Myocardial infarction: Electrocardiographic differential diagnosis*, ed 4, St Louis, Mosby, 1991.

QRS Complexes

Amplitude: Normal if pleural effusion absent. QRS complexes may be low voltage (amplitude) if pleural effusion is present. If pleural effusion is severe, cardiac tamponade may occur, causing the QRS complexes to alternate between normal and low voltage, coincident with respiration (electrical alternans).

Abnormal Q Waves/QS Complexes: Absent.

ST Segments: ST segments are usually elevated in most, if not all, leads except leads aVR and V_1, because pericarditis usually affects the entire myocardial surface of the heart. In lead aVR, the ST segment is either normal or slightly depressed. Reciprocal ST-segment depression usually is not present. The ST segments return to normal as the pericarditis resolves.

T Waves: Elevated during the acute phase of pericarditis in the leads with ST-segment elevation. The elevated T waves become inverted as the pericarditis resolves.

QT Intervals: Normal.

Location of Pericarditis	Leads with ST-Segment Elevation
Anterior	V_2-V_4
Lateral	I, aVL, V_5-V_6
Inferior	II, III, aVF
Generalized	I, II, III, aVL, aVF, V_2-V_6

ELECTROLYTE IMBALANCE

Hyperkalemia

P Waves: Begin to flatten out and become wider at a serum potassium level of approximately 6.5 mEq/L and disappear at levels of approximately 7 to 9 mEq/L.

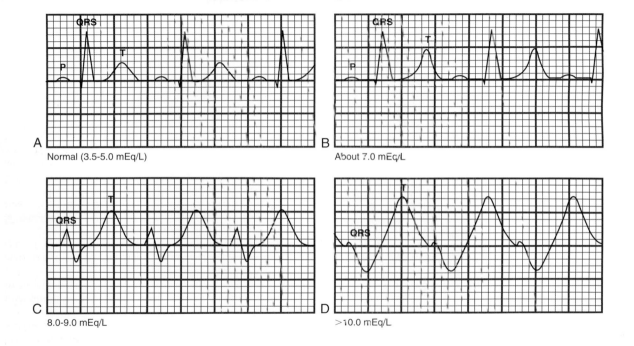

A
Normal (3.5-5.0 mEq/L)

B
About 7.0 mEq/L

C
8.0-9.0 mEq/L

D
>10.0 mEq/L

PR Intervals: May be normal or prolonged, greater than 0.20 second. Absent when the P waves disappear.

QRS Complexes: Begin to widen at serum potassium levels of approximately 6.0 to 6.5 mEq/L, becoming significantly slurred and abnormally widened beyond 0.12 second at 10 mEq/L. At this point they "merge" with the following T waves, resulting in a "sine wave" QRS-ST-T pattern.

ST Segments: Disappear at a serum potassium level of approximately 6 mEq/L.

T Waves: Become typically tall and peaked with a narrower than normal base at serum potassium levels of approximately 5.5 to 6.5 mEq/L. Earliest T wave changes are best seen in leads II, III, and V_2-V_4.

Cause of Hyperkalemia: Excess of serum potassium above the normal levels of 3.5 to 5.0 mEq/L. The most common causes of hyperkalemia are the following:
- Kidney failure
- Certain diuretics (e.g., triamterene)

Associated Dysrhythmias

- Sinus arrest (may occur at a serum potassium level of approximately 7.5 mEq/L)
- Cardiac standstill (may occur at serum potassium levels of approximately 10 to 12 mEq/L)
- Ventricular fibrillation (may occur at serum potassium levels of approximately 10 to 12 mEq/L)

Hypokalemia

Hypokalemia

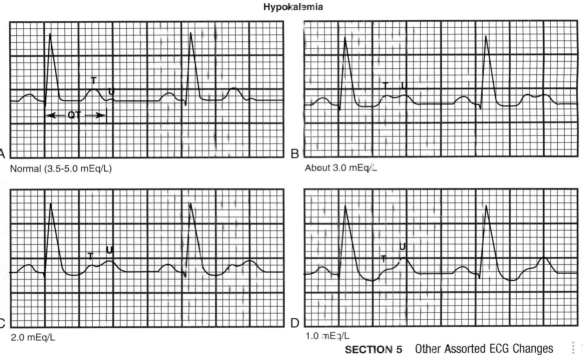

A Normal (3.5-5.0 mEq/L)

B About 3.0 mEq/L

C 2.0 mEq/L

D 1.0 mEq/L

P Waves: Become typically tall and symmetrically peaked, with an amplitude of >2.5 mm in leads II, III, and aVF at a serum potassium level of 2 mEq/L (pseudo P pulmonale).

QRS Complexes: Begin to widen at a serum potassium level of approximately 3.0 mEq/L.

ST Segments: May become depressed by 1 mm or more.

T Waves: Begin to flatten at a serum potassium level of approximately 3.0 mEq/L and continue to become smaller as the U waves increase in size. The T waves may either merge with the U waves or become inverted.

U Waves: Begin to increase in size, becoming as tall ("prominent") as the T waves at a serum potassium level of approximately 3.0 mEq/L and, at approximately 2 mEq/L, becoming taller than the T waves. The U waves reach "giant" size and fuse with the T waves at 1 mEq/L.

QT Intervals: May appear to be prolonged when the U waves become prominent and fuse with the T waves but actually remain normal.

Cause of Hypokalemia: Deficiency of serum potassium below the normal levels of 3.5 to 5.0 mEq/L. Causes of hypokalemia are the following:
- Loss of potassium in body fluids through vomiting, gastric suction, and excessive use of diuretics (the most common causes)
- Low serum magnesium levels (hypomagnesemia)

The ECG characteristics of hypomagnesemia, incidentally, resemble those of hypokalemia.

Associated Dysrhythmias: Ventricular dysrhythmias, including torsades de pointes (may occur in hypokalemia in the presence of digitalis)

Hypercalcemia

Hypercalcemia and hypocalcemia

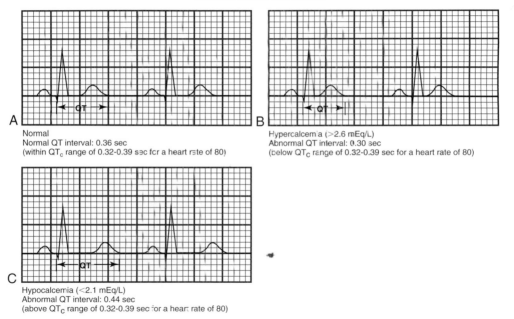

A
Normal
Normal QT interval: 0.36 sec
(within QT$_c$ range of 0.32-0.39 sec for a heart rate of 80)

B
Hypercalcemia (>2.6 mEq/L)
Abnormal QT interval: 0.30 sec
(below QT$_c$ range of 0.32-0.39 sec for a heart rate of 80)

C
Hypocalcemia (<2.1 mEq/L)
Abnormal QT interval: 0.44 sec
(above QT$_c$ range of 0.32-0.39 sec for a heart rate of 80)

QT Intervals: Shorter than normal for the heart rate.

Cause of Hypercalcemia: Excess of serum calcium above the normal levels of 2.1 to 2.6 mEq/L (or 4.25 to 5.25 mg/100 mL). Common causes of hypercalcemia include the following:

- Adrenal insufficiency
- Hyperparathyroidism
- Immobilization
- Kidney failure
- Malignancy
- Sarcoidosis
- Thyrotoxicosis
- Vitamin A and D intoxication

Hypocalcemia

ST Segments: Prolonged.

QT Intervals: Prolonged beyond the normal limits for the heart rate because of the prolonged ST segments.

Cause of Hypocalcemia: Deficiency of serum calcium below the normal levels of 2.1 to 2.6 mEq/L (or 4.25 to 5.25 mg/100 mL). Common causes of hypocalcemia include the following:

- Chronic steatorrhea
- Diuretics (such as furosemide or ethacrynic acid)
- Respiratory alkalosis and hyperventilation
- Osteomalacia in adults and rickets in children
- Pregnancy
- Hypoparathyroidism
- Hypomagnesemia (possibly because of release of parathyroid hormone)

DRUG EFFECT

Digitalis

PR Intervals: Prolonged over 0.2 second.

ST Segments: Depressed 1 mm or more in many of the leads, with a characteristic "scooped-out" appearance.

T Waves: May be flattened, inverted, or biphasic.

QT Intervals: Shorter than normal for the heart rate.

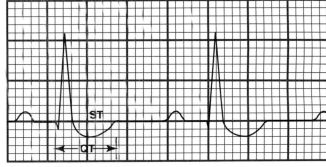

Abnormal QT interval: 0.30 sec
(below QT_c range of 0.32-0.39 sec for a heart rate of 80)

Effects of Digitalis Toxicity: Excessive administration of digitalis may cause excitatory and inhibitory effects on the heart and its electrical conduction system.

Excitatory effects include the following:
- Premature atrial complexes
- Atrial tachycardia with or without block
- Nonparoxysmal junctional tachycardia
- Premature ventricular complexes
- Ventricular tachycardia
- Ventricular fibrillation

Inhibitory effects include the following:
- Sinus bradycardia
- Sinoatrial (SA) exit block
- Atrioventricular (AV) block

Procainamide

PR Intervals: May be prolonged.

QRS Complexes
Duration: May be increased beyond 0.12 second, a sign of
procainamide toxicity.
R waves: May be decreased in amplitude.

ST Segments: May be depressed 1 mm or more.

T Waves: May be decreased in amplitude and occasionally
widened and notched because of the appearance of a U wave.

QT Intervals: May occasionally be prolonged beyond the normal
limits for the heart rate, a sign of procainamide toxicity.

Effects of Procainamide Toxicity: Excessive administration
of procainamide may cause excitatory and inhibitory effects on the
heart and its electrical conduction system.

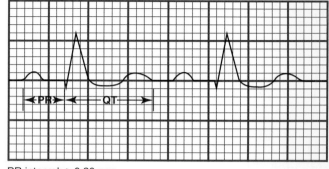

PR interval: >0.20 sec
QT interval: Prolonged, 0.45 sec
(above QT_C range of 0.32-0.39 sec for a heart rate of 80)
QRS complex: Widened, >0.12 sec

Excitatory effects include the following:
- Premature ventricular complexes
- Torsades de pointes (occurrence less common than in quinidine toxicity)
- Ventricular fibrillation

Inhibitory effects include the following:
- Depression of myocardial contractility, which may cause hypotension and congestive heart failure
- AV block
- Ventricular asystole

PULMONARY DISEASE

Pulmonary Embolism (Acute)

Pulmonary Embolism (Acute)

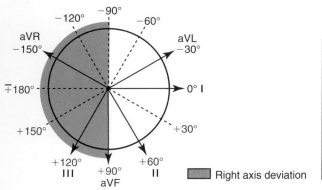

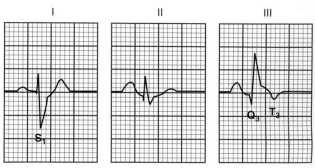

P Waves: Right atrial enlargement may be present (P pulmonale).

QRS Complexes
Q Waves: Abnormal Q waves in lead III.
S Waves: Deep S waves in lead I.

T Waves: Inverted T waves in lead III.

ST Segments/T Waves: Right ventricular "strain" pattern may be present in leads V_1-V_3.

QRS Pattern: An $S_1Q_3T_3$ pattern may occur acutely. In addition, a right bundle branch block may also occur.

QRS Axis: Greater than +90°.

Associated Dysrhythmias: Sinus tachycardia.

Chronic Cor Pulmonale

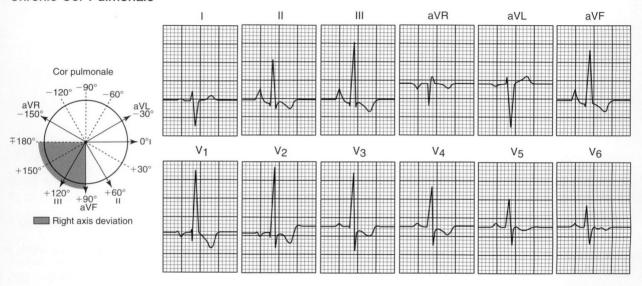

P Waves: Right atrial enlargement present (P pulmonale).

QRS Complexes: Right ventricular hypertrophy present.

ST Segments/T Waves: Right ventricular "strain" pattern in leads V_1-V_3.

QRS Axis: Greater than +90°.

Associated Dysrhythmias
- Premature atrial complexes
- Wandering atrial pacemaker
- Multifocal atrial tachycardia
- Atrial flutter
- Atrial fibrillation

Early Repolarization

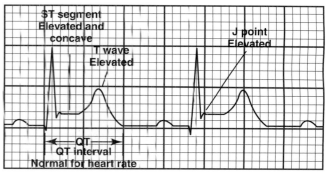

QRS Complexes: Abnormal Q waves usually absent.

ST Segments: Elevated by approximately 1 to 3 mm or more in leads I, II, and aVF and in the precordial leads V_2-V_6. May be depressed in lead aVR.

T Waves: Usually normal.

Cause of Early Repolarization: A normal ECG variant that occurs in normal healthy people, commonly in young persons and sometimes in the elderly.

Hypothermia

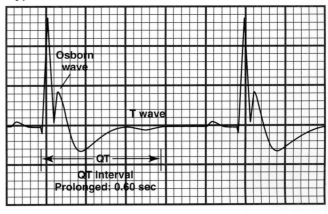

PR Intervals: May occasionally be prolonged, greater than 0.20 second.

QRS Complexes: May occasionally be abnormally wide, greater than 0.12 second. Typically followed by an Osborn wave

QT Intervals: Corrected QT interval (QTc interval) may occasionally be prolonged.

Osborn Wave: A narrow positive deflection at the junction of the QRS complex and the ST segment. Typically seen in the leads facing the left ventricle (leads I, II, III, aVL, aVF, and V_3-V_6).

Associated Dysrhythmias
- Sinus bradycardia
- Junctional dysrhythmias
- Ventricular dysrhythmias

PREEXCITATION SYNDROMES

Ventricular Preexcitation

Preexcitation Syndromes

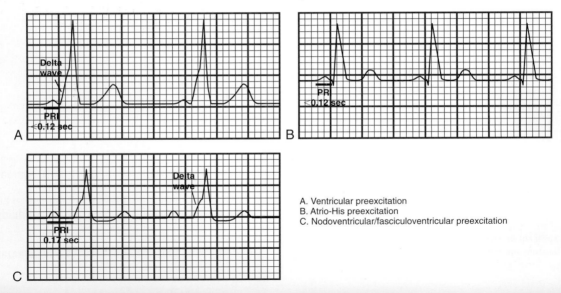

A. Ventricular preexcitation
B. Atrio-His preexcitation
C. Nodoventricular/fasciculoventricular preexcitation

PR Intervals: Abnormally short, usually less than 0.12 second; between 0.09 and 0.12 second.

QRS Complexes: Duration greater than 0.10 second. A delta wave is present.

Atrio-His Preexcitation

PR Intervals: Abnormally short, usually less than 0.12 second.

QRS Complexes: Duration normal, 0.10 second or less. A delta wave is not present.

Nodoventricular/Fasciculoventricular Preexcitation

PR Intervals: Normal, 0.12 second or greater.

QRS Complexes: Duration greater than 0.10 second. A delta wave is present.

Cause of Preexcitation Syndromes

- **Ventricular Preexcitation.** Aberrant conduction of an electrical impulse through an abnormal accessory AV pathway that bypasses the AV junction, resulting in premature depolarization of the ventricles and an abnormally short PR interval.
- **Atrio-His Preexcitation.** Aberrant conduction of an electrical impulse through abnormal atrio-His fibers that bypass the AV node, resulting in an abnormally short PR interval but normal depolarization of the ventricles.
- **Nodoventricular/Fasciculoventricular Preexcitation.** Aberrant conduction of an electrical impulse through abnormal nodoventricular or fasciculoventricular fibers that bypass the entire bundle of His or the distal part of it, respectively, resulting in premature depolarization of the ventricles and a normal PR interval.

Brugada Syndrome

QRS Complexes: The QRS complexes in V_1-V_3 resemble a right bundle branch block without the typical RSR′ pattern.

ST Segments: The ST segments associated with the abnormal QRS complexes in the precordial leads have a non-ischemic elevation pattern (no reciprocal changes).

Brugada Pattern

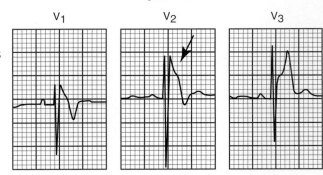

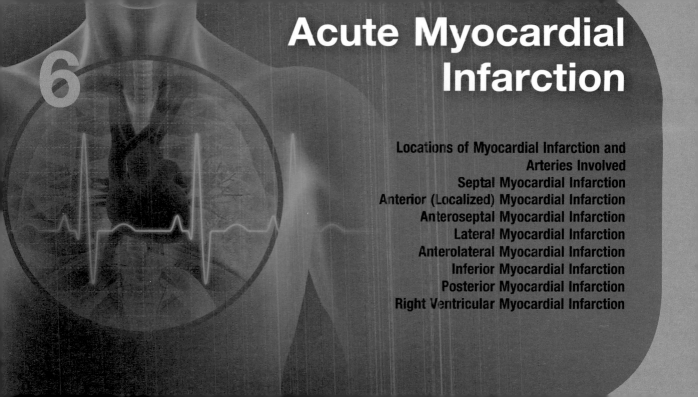

Acute Myocardial Infarction

6

Locations of Myocardial Infarction and Arteries Involved

Septal MI

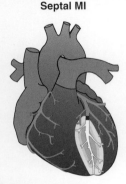

Arteries involved:
Left anterior descending artery
Septal perforator branches

Localized anterior MI

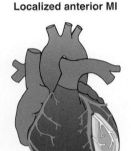

Left anterior descending artery
Diagonal branches

Anteroseptal MI

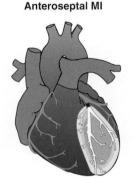

Left anterior descending artery
Septal perforator branches
Diagonal branches

Lateral MI

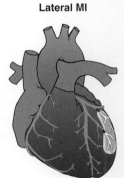

Left anterior descending artery
Diagonal branches
Left circumflex artery
Anterolateral marginal branch

Anterolateral MI

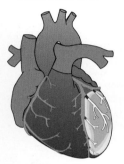

Exensive anterior MI

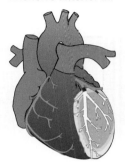

Inferior MI

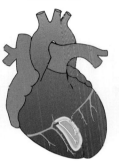

Posterior MI

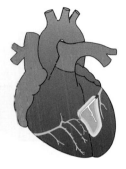

Right ventricular MI

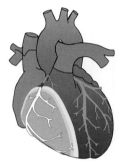

Arteries involved:

Left anterior descending artery
  Diagonal branches
Left circumflex artery
  Anterolateral marginal branch

Left anterior descending artery
Left circumflex
  Anterolateral marginal branch

Right coronary (or left circumflex) artery
  Posterior left ventricular branches

Distal left circumflex artery and/or its posterolateral branch

Right coronary artery

Septal Myocardial Infarction

Early

Phase 1: First Few Hours (0 to 2 Hours)

ECG Changes:

- In facing leads V_1-V_2:
  - Absence of normal "septal" r waves in leads V_1-V_2, resulting in QS waves in these leads
  - ST-segment elevation with tall T waves in leads V_1-V_2
- In leads I, II, III, aVF, and V_4-V_6:
  - Absence of normal "septal" q waves where normally present in leads I, II, III, aVF, and V_4-V_6
- In opposite leads II, III, and aVF:
  - No significant ECG changes in leads II, III, and aVF

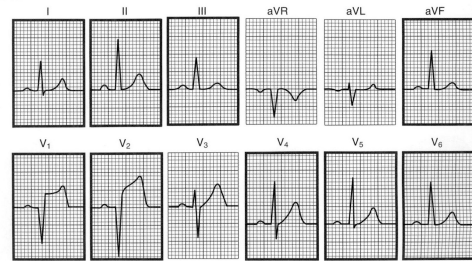

Phase 2: First Day (2 to 24 Hours)
ECG Changes:
- In facing leads V_1-V_2:
  - Maximal ST-segment elevation in leads V_1-V_2

Late

Phase 3: Second and Third Days (24 to 72 Hours)
ECG Changes:
- In facing leads V_1-V_2:
  - QS complexes with T wave inversion in leads V_1-V_2
  - Return of ST segments to baseline in leads V_1-V_2
- In opposite leads II, III, and aVF:
  - No significant ECG changes in leads II, III, and aVF

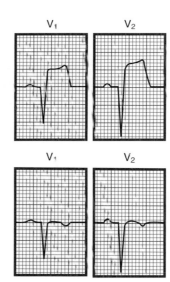

Anterior (Localized) Myocardial Infarction

Early

Phase 1: First Few
Hours (0 to 2 Hours)
ECG Changes:

- In facing leads V_3-V_4:
  - ST-segment
    elevation with tall
    T waves and
    taller than
    normal R waves
    in leads V_3-V_4
- In opposite leads II,
  III, and aVF:
  - No significant
    ECG changes in
    leads II, III, and
    aVF

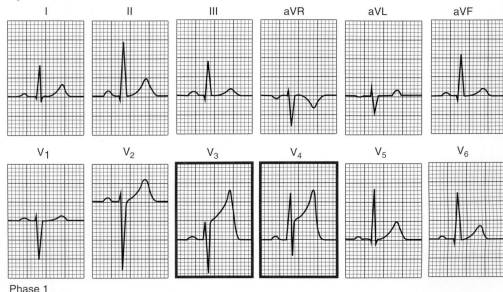

Phase 1

Phase 2: First Day (2 to 24 Hours)

ECG Changes:

- In facing leads V_3-V_4:
  - Minimally abnormal Q waves in leads V_3-V_4
  - Maximal ST-segment elevation in leads V_3-V_4

Late

Phase 3: Second and Third Days (24 to 72 Hours)

ECG Changes:

- In facing leads V_3-V_4:
  - QS complexes with T wave inversion in leads V_3-V_4
  - Return of ST segments to baseline in leads V_3-V_4
- In opposite leads II, III, and aVF:
  - No significant ECG changes in leads II, III, and aVF

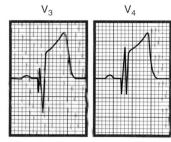

Phase 2

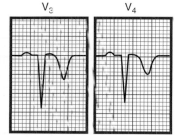

Phase 3

Anteroseptal Myocardial Infarction

Early

Phase 1: First Few Hours
(0 to 2 Hours)
ECG Changes:

- In facing leads V_1-V_4:
  - Absence of normal "septal" r waves in leads V_1-V_2, resulting in QS waves in these leads
  - ST segment elevation with tall T waves in leads V_1-V_4
  - Taller than normal R waves in leads V_3-V_4
- In leads I, II, III, aVF, and V_4-V_6:
  - Absence of normal "septal" q waves

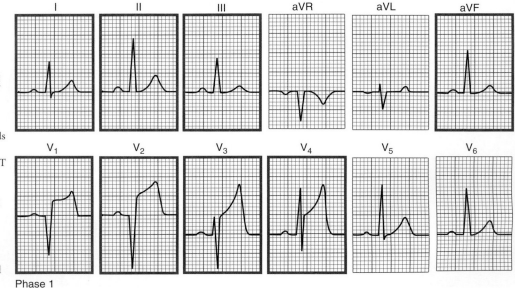

Phase 1

where normally present in leads I, II, III, aVF, and V_4-V_6
- In opposite leads II, III, and aVF:
  - No significant ECG changes in leads II, III, and aVF

Phase 2: First Day (2 to 24 Hours)
ECG Changes:
- In facing leads V_1-V_4:
  - Minimally abnormal Q waves in leads V_3-V_4
  - Maximal ST-segment elevation in leads V_1-V_4

Late

Phase 3: Second and Third Days (24 to 72 Hours)
ECG Changes:
- In facing leads V_1-V_4:
  - QS complexes with T wave inversion in leads V_1-V_4
  - Return of ST segments to baseline in leads V_1-V_4
- In opposite leads II, III, and aVF:
  - No significant ECG changes in leads II, III, and aVF

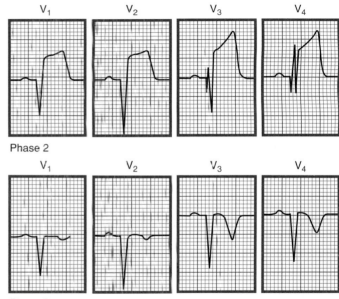

Phase 2

Phase 3

Lateral Myocardial Infarction
Early

Phase 1: First Few
Hours (0 to 2 Hours)
ECG Changes:
- In facing leads I,
  aVL, and V_5-V_6:
  - ST-segment
    elevation with tall
    T waves and
    taller than
    normal R waves
    in leads I, aVL,
    and lead V_5 or V_6
    or both
- In opposite leads II,
  III, and aVF:
  - ST-segment
    depression in
    leads II, III, and
    aVF

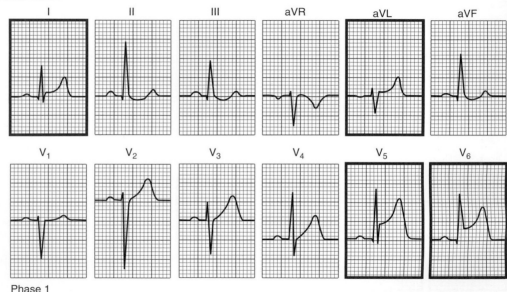

Phase 1

Phase 2: First Day (2 to 24 Hours)

ECG Changes:

- In facing leads I, aVL, and V_5-V_6:
  - Minimally abnormal Q waves in leads I and aVL and lead V_5 or V_6 or both
  - Maximal ST-segment elevation in leads I and aVL and lead V_5 or V_6 or both

Late

Phase 3: Second and Third Days (24 to 72 Hours)

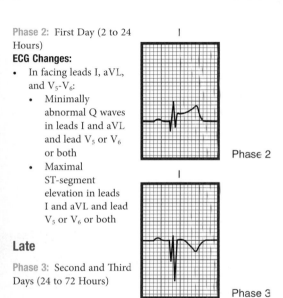

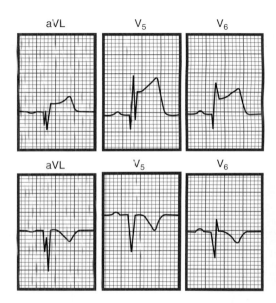

ECG Changes:

- In facing leads I, aVL, and V_5-V_6:
  - Abnormal Q waves and small R waves with T wave inversion in leads I and aVL
  - QS waves or complexes and decreased or absent R waves with T wave inversion in lead V_5 or V_6 or both
  - Return of ST segments to baseline

- In opposite leads II, III, and aVF:
  - Tall T waves in leads II, III, and aVF
  - Return of ST segments to baseline

Anterolateral Myocardial Infarction

Early

Phase 1: First Few Hours
(0 to 2 Hours)
ECG Changes:

- In facing leads I, aVL,
  and V_3-V_6:
  - ST-segment
    elevation with tall
    T waves and taller
    than normal R
    waves in leads I,
    aVL, and V_3-V_6
- In opposite leads II,
  III, and aVF:
  - ST-segment
    depression in
    leads II, III, and
    aVF

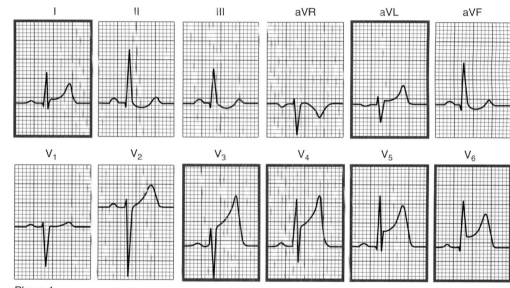

Phase 1

Phase 2: First Day (2 to 24 Hours)
ECG Changes:
- In facing leads I, aVL, and V_3-V_6:
  - Minimally abnormal Q waves in leads I, aVL, and V_3-V_6
  - Maximal ST-segment elevation in leads I, aVL, and V_3-V_6

Late

Phase 3: Second and Third Days (24 to 72 Hours)
ECG Changes:
- In facing leads I, aVL, and V_3-V_6:

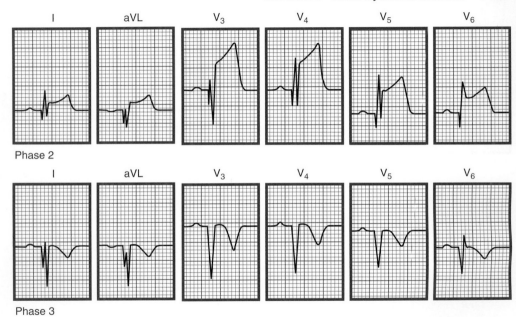

- Abnormal Q waves and small R waves with T wave inversion in leads I and aVL
- QS waves or complexes and decreased or absent R waves with T wave inversion in leads V_3-V_6
- Return of ST segments to baseline

- In opposite leads II, III, and aVF:
  - Tall T waves in leads II, III, and aVF
  - Return of ST segments to baseline

Inferior Myocardial Infarction
Early

Phase 1: First Few Hours
(0 to 2 Hours)
ECG Changes:

- In facing leads II, III, and aVF:
  - ST-segment elevation with tall T waves and taller than normal R waves in leads II, III, and aVF
- In opposite leads I and aVL:
  - ST-segment depression in leads I and aVL

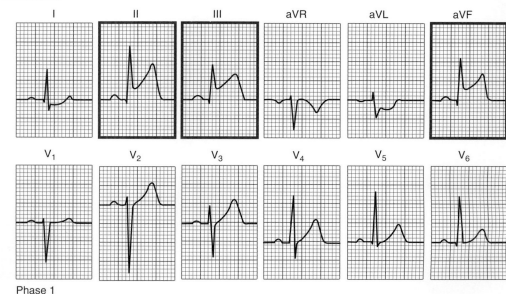

Phase 1

Phase 2: First Day (2 to 24 Hours)
ECG Changes:

- In facing leads II, III, and aVF:
    - Minimally abnormal Q waves in leads II, III, and aVF
    - Maximal ST-segment elevation in leads II, III, and aVF

Late

Phase 3: Second and Third Days (24 to 72 Hours)
ECG Changes:

- In facing leads II, III, and aVF:
    - QS waves or complexes and decreased or absent R waves with T wave inversion in leads II, III, and aVF
    - Return of ST segments to baseline
- In opposite leads I and aVL:
    - Tall T waves in leads I and aVL
    - Return of ST segments to baseline

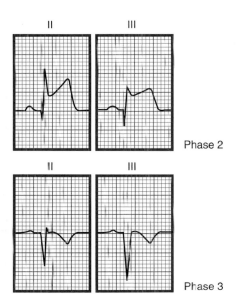

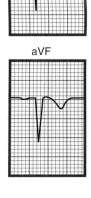

Posterior Myocardial Infarction

Early

Phase 1: First Few Hours
(0 to 2 Hours)
ECG Changes:

- In facing leads: No
  facing leads present.
- In opposite leads
  V_1-V_4:
  - ST-segment
    depression in leads
    V_1-V_4
  - T wave inversion
    in V_1 and
    sometimes V_2

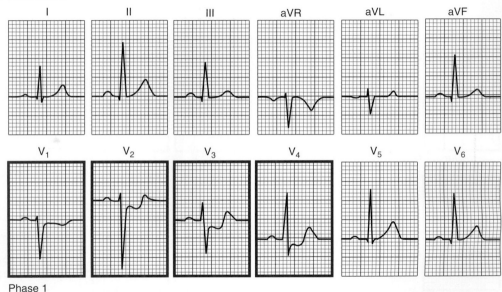

Phase 1

Phase 2: First Day (2 to 24 Hours)
ECG Changes:
- In facing leads: No facing leads present.
- In opposite leads V_1-V_4:
  - Maximal ST-segment depression in leads V_1-V_4

Late

Phase 3: Second and Third Days (24 to 72 Hours)
ECG Changes:
- In facing leads: No facing leads present.
- In opposite leads V_1-V_4:
  - Large R waves with tall T waves in leads V_1-V_4; the R waves in lead V_1 are tall and wide (>0.04 second in width) with slurring and notching
  - Smaller than normal S waves in lead V_1, resulting in an R/S ratio of >1 in this lead
  - Return of ST segments to baseline in leads V_1-V_4

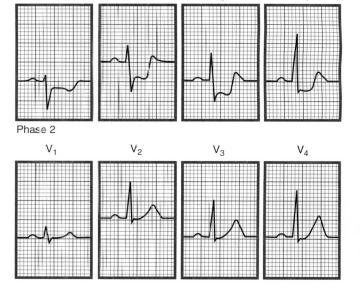

Phase 2

Phase 3

Right Ventricular Myocardial Infarction

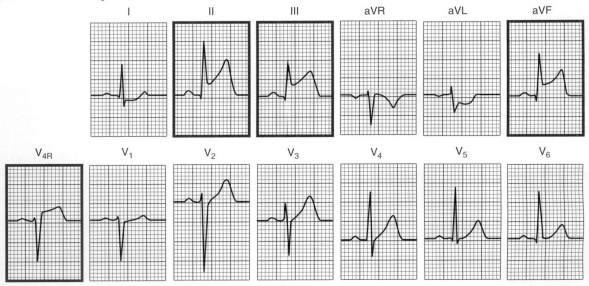

Early

Phase 1: First Few Hours (0 to 2 Hours)
ECG Changes:
- In facing leads II, III, aVF, and V_{4R}:
  - ST-segment elevation in leads II, III, aVF, and V_{4R}
  - Tall T waves and taller than normal R waves in leads II, III, and aVF
- In opposite leads I and aVL:
  - ST-segment depression in leads I and aVL

Phase 2: First Day (2 to 24 Hours)
ECG Changes:
- In facing leads II, III, aVF, and V_{4R}:
  - Minimally abnormal Q waves in leads II, III, and aVF
  - Maximal ST-segment elevation in leads II, III, and aVF
  - ST-segment elevation in lead V_{4R}, but ST segment may be normal

Late

Phase 3: Second and Third Days (24 to 72 Hours)
ECG Changes:
- In facing leads II, III, aVF, and V_{4R}:
  - QS waves or complexes and decreased or absent R waves in leads II, III, and aVF
  - T wave inversion in leads II, III, aVF, and V_{4R}
  - Return of ST segments to baseline
- In opposite leads I and aVL:
  - Tall T waves in leads I and aVL
  - Return of ST segments to baseline

Management of Acute Coronary Syndromes

7

Signs and Symptoms of Acute Coronary Syndromes

Pain is the most common symptom, appearing in 70% to 80% of the patients with acute myocardial infarction (MI) who are not in shock or cardiac arrest. One or more of the following signs and symptoms frequently accompany the pain of acute coronary syndrome (ACS), depending on the degree of heart failure present and whether a dysrhythmia is present. It is important to note that many of these signs and symptoms may be present even in the absence of pain, as in a so-called *silent acute MI*. The finding of any one or more of the following symptoms should lead one to suspect acute MI, especially if the patient is middle-aged or older.

Symptoms in Acute Coronary Syndrome

- **General and neurological symptoms.** Anxiety and apprehension, extreme fatigue and weakness, restlessness, and agitation, with a fear of impending death (or a sense of impending doom) are common. Lightheadedness or dizziness, confusion, disorientation, drowsiness, or loss of consciousness may also be present.
- **Cardiovascular symptoms.** Chest pain and palpitations or "skipping of the heart" are usually present in the majority of the patients.

- **Respiratory symptoms.** Dyspnea is common, often accompanied by a sensation of suffocation; a tight, constricted feeling in the chest; and even pain on breathing. Wheezing; spasmodic coughing, often productive of copious, frothy sputum, frequently pink- or blood-tinged (hemoptysis).
- **Gastrointestinal symptoms.** Nausea, with or without vomiting, and a loss of appetite (anorexia) are common. If gastrointestinal symptoms are present, and especially if the chest pain radiates to the epigastrium, the patient often misinterprets the symptoms as being those of indigestion and ignores them.

Signs in Acute Coronary Syndrome

- **General appearance and neurological signs.** The patient may be alert and oriented initially but restless, anxious, and apprehensive or confused and disoriented. The patient may become drowsy and unresponsive and then lose consciousness and convulse.
- **Vital Signs**
  - **Pulse.** The pulse is usually rapid, over 100/bpm (tachycardia), but may be 60 to 100/bpm (normal) or less than 60/bpm (bradycardia). The rhythm may be regular or irregular. The force of the pulse may be normal, strong, and full; or if hypotension or shock is present, it may be weak and thready.

- **Respirations.** The respirations are typically greater than 16/min (tachypnea) and shallow, but may be 12 to 16/min (normal, eupnea) or less. The rhythm of the respirations may be regular or irregular; their depth may be normal, shallow, or deep. The respirations may be labored and noisy or gasping. Hyperpnea may be present. The accessory muscles of respiration may be prominent during breathing if severe pulmonary congestion and edema are present.
- **Blood pressure.** The systolic blood pressure may be normal, elevated (>140 mm Hg), or low (<90 mm Hg) if hypotension or shock is present.
- **Skin.** The skin is usually pale, cold, sweaty, and clammy. Cyanosis of the skin, fingernail beds, and mucous membranes is present if pulmonary congestion and edema is present. Skin is mottled bluish-red if shock is present. The lips may be normal in color, pale, or cyanotic. Delayed capillary refill indicated poor perfusion.
- **Veins.** With the patient lying flat or propped up at a 45-degree angle, the neck veins may be normal, moderately distended (in left heart failure and mild right heart failure), markedly distended and pulsating (in severe right heart failure), or collapsed (in hypotension or shock). The superficial veins of the body may be normal, distended, or collapsed.
- **Cardiovascular signs.** The heart sounds are usually distant. A fourth heart sound (S_4) is non-diagnostic, whereas the presence of a third heart sound (S_3) indicates left ventricular dysfunction. Friction rubs indicate myocardial inflammation
- **Respiratory signs.** Breathing may be normal or labored and noisy. Wheezing; dry, coarse rattling in the throat; spasmodic coughing, with expectoration of frothy sputum, often pink- or blood-tinged (hemoptysis). Dullness to percussion may be present over one or both lungs, particularly at the bases of the lungs posteriorly. On auscultation, the breath sounds may be normal, decreased, or absent. Rales, wheezes, rhonchi, and possibly loud gurgling or bubbling sounds may be present at one or both bases of the lungs only or up to the scapulae posteriorly or throughout the lungs.
- **Body tissue edema.** Pitting edema in the lower extremities, particularly in the ankles and feet and in front of the tibia (pedal and pretibial edema), lower part of the back over the spine (presacral edema), and abdominal wall may be present in right heart failure. If the tissues of the entire body are edematous, anasarca is present.

Risk Stratification

Once the history and physical examination is completed, the clinician should be able with a fair degree of accuracy to determine the likelihood that the patient's symptoms are consistent with an ACS. It is important to perform this risk assessment at this point before relying solely on the electrocardiogram (ECG) and cardiac enzymes for the following reason: (1) the ECG may be nondiagnostic and/or (2) the cardiac enzymes may not be available or the patient may need to be transferred to definitive care. Box 7-1 provides a method of assessing the likelihood that the pain is consistent with ACS. At this point, a diagnostic 12-lead ECG should be performed and the indications of STEMI and non-STEMI assessed.

The 12-Lead ECG

The 12-lead ECG is critical to proceeding with the workup of the suspected ACS. If the ECG shows diagnostic ST elevation in contiguous leads as discussed in Chapter 17 of the main text, then the diagnosis of STEMI is made. If ST depression and T wave inversion are present, then non-STEMI is more likely; however, a posterior wall MI must be considered. In the absence of ST segment changes, the working diagnosis is unstable angina. Until the levels of the cardiac markers are known, the patient is now in the unstable angina/NSTEMI category. However, recognizing the limitations of the 12-lead ECG will provide the astute clinician more confidence in the diagnosis of ACS.

> **BOX 7-1 Reasons Patients Delay Seeking Medical Attention for Symptoms of ACS**
>
> - They expected a more dramatic presentation
> - Thought symptoms were not serious or would go away
> - Tried "self-treatment," antacids, their own nitroglycerin, aspirin, etc.
> - Attributed symptoms to chronic conditions such as arthritis, muscle spasm, etc.
> - Lacked awareness of benefits of reperfusion treatments or importance of 9-1-1
> - Fear of embarrassment if "false alarm," thought they needed "permission" to come office
> - Did not perceive themselves at risk
>   - Young and healthy (especially men)
>   - Women
>   - Under a doctor's care or making lifestyle changes for risk factors
>
> Based on findings from Finnegan JR Jr, Meischke H, Zapka JG, et al: Patient delay in seeking care for heart attack symptoms: findings from focus groups conducted in five U.S. regions, *Prev Med* 31:205-13, 2000.

The diagnosis of myocardial infarction is confirmed with cardiac markers in more than 90% of patients with ST-segment elevation. Up to 25% of patients with NSTEMI and elevated CK-MB develop Q-wave myocardial infarctions whereas the remaining 75% have non–Q-wave MIs. One to 6% of patient with a completely normal ECG and chest pain are eventually diagnosed with NSTEMI and at least 4% will have unstable angina.

In the event the initial ECG is nondiagnostic, obtaining serial 12-leads ECGs or monitoring the patient with continuous ST-segment deviation monitoring allows the clinician to detect subtle changes in the ECG, which can confirm the diagnosis and appropriately alter the therapy. Obtaining 12-lead ECGs when the patient is symptomatic is significantly more accurate in detecting ST changes if the pain is secondary to an ACS.

ACUTE CORONARY SYNDROME MANAGEMENT

A. Initial Assessment and Management of a Patient with Chest Pain

Prehospital/Emergency Department

- Administer oxygen 2-4 L/min via nasal cannula or 100% NRB if signs of respiratory distress.
- Quickly assess the patient's circulatory status while obtaining the vital signs, including level of consciousness, and repeat as the situation requires and circumstances permit.
- Start monitoring the ECG for significant dysrhythmias.
- Start an intravenous (IV) line with either normal saline (NS) or 5% dextrose in water (D5W) to keep the vein open (TKO) to administer medications.
- While performing these steps, obtain a brief history and physical examination to determine the cause of the chest pain.
- Obtain a 12-lead ECG (plus lead V_{4R}, if indicated), using an ECG monitor with or without computerized ECG interpretation, and, if appropriate, transmit the 12-lead ECG and/or the computerized

ECG interpretation to the base hospital for physician interpretation.
- Determine whether
  - Normal ECG
  - Nondiagnostic ECG
  - ST depression
  - ST elevation MI (Criteria A)
- Evaluate the ECG. If any of the following ECG changes are present, the ECG is diagnostic of an acute MI:
  - ST-segment elevation of ≥1 mm in two or more contiguous leads (indicative of an acute anterior, lateral, inferior, or right ventricular MI)
  - ST-segment depression of ≥1 mm in two or more contiguous precordial leads (indicative of an acute posterior MI)
  - New or presumably new LBBB on the ECG is diagnostic of an acute MI

B. Initial Treatment and Assessment of Suspected Acute MI
Prehospital/Emergency Department
- Administer a **chewable aspirin** 162-325 mg.
- If chest pain is present:
  - Administer **nitroglycerin** 0.4 mg by sublingual tablet or lingual aerosol if the patient's systolic blood pressure is 100 mm Hg or greater. Administer with the patient sitting or lying down. If hypotension does not occur, repeat approximately every 5 minutes as necessary, for a total dose of three tablets or three lingual aerosol applications.

  AND

  If nitroglycerin is not effective after the third dose or the pain is severe:
  - Administer **morphine sulfate** 2-4 mg IV slowly over 3-5 minutes and repeat in 5-10 minutes as necessary, up to a total dose of 10-20 mg.
- Start an IV infusion of **nitroglycerin** at a rate of 5 µg/min and increase the rate of infusion by 5 µg/min every 5-10 minutes until one of the following occurs, at which time stop increasing the infusion rate and continue it at its current rate:
  - The chest pain is relieved
  - The mean arterial blood pressure drops by 10% in a normotensive patient
  - The mean arterial blood pressure drops by 30% in a hypertensive patient

  AND

If the mean arterial blood pressure drops below 80 mm Hg or the systolic blood pressure drops below 90 mm Hg at any time:

- ○ Slow or temporarily stop the IV infusion of nitroglycerin
- If the patient is apprehensive and anxious but has little or no pain consider an anxiolytic:
  - ○ Administer **diazepam** 2.5-5 mg IV slowly, or **lorazepam** 0.5-1 mg IV slowly.
- If nausea or vomiting is present:
  - ○ Administer **promethazine hydrochloride** 12.5-25 mg IV or **ondansetron** 4 mg IV.
- If STEMI is confirmed
  - ○ Proceed immediately to Section C, *Reperfusion Therapy: STEMI Protocol*

C. Reperfusion Therapy: STEMI protocol

Once the 12-lead ECG is obtained and meets STEMI criteria, a decision must be made as to the most appropriate reperfusion therapy.

If PCI can be accomplished within 90 minutes proceed to Primary PCI

PRIMARY PCI

Emergency Department

- Administer an anticoagulant such as LMW heparin (enoxaparin) or unfractionated heparin.
  - ○ Administer **enoxaparin** 30 mg IV followed in 15 minutes by 1 mg/kg **enoxaparin** subcutaneously.

  OR

  Administer a 60 U/kg bolus of unfractionated **heparin** IV (maximum 4000 U bolus for patients ≥70 kg followed by a 12 U/kg/hr unfractionated **heparin** IV infusion (maximum 1000 U/hr for patients >70 kg) to maintain an aPTT of 50-70 seconds.
- Consider the administration of a **GP IIb/IIIa receptor inhibitor** for patients younger than 75 with extensive anterior MIs and minimal risk of bleeding.
  - ○ Administer **abciximab** 0.25 mg/kg IV **AND** start an **abciximab** infusion at 0.125 µg/kg/min.

  OR

  - ○ Administer **eptifibatide** 180 µg/kg IV **AND** start an **eptifibatide** infusion at 2 µg/kg/min.
- Move rapidly to catheterization lab

- **IF PCI cannot be performed within 90 minutes**
  - Determine patient's eligibility for fibrinolytic therapy (Box 7-2)
  - Determine whether any absolute contraindications for fibrinolytic therapy exist (Box 7-3)
  - Proceed to fibrinolytic administration

FIBRINOLYTIC ADMINISTRATION

Emergency Department

If acute MI is confirmed and no contraindications to fibrinolytic therapy are present:

- Administer a fibrinolytic agent.
  - Administer **reteplase** 10 units IV over 2 minutes and repeat in 30 minutes.

      OR
  - Administer **tenecteplase** 30-50 mg IV over 5 seconds based on the patient's weight as indicated in Table 7-1.
- Administer an anticoagulant such as LMW heparin (enoxaparin) or unfractionated heparin.
  - Administer a 30-mg bolus of **enoxaparin** IV followed in 15 minutes by 1 mg/kg enoxaparin subcutaneously.

      OR

TABLE 7-1 **Tenecteplase Dosage Table**

Patient Weight	<60 kg	60 to <70 kg	70 to <80 kg	80 to <90 kg	≥90 kg
TNK-tPA (mg)	30 mg	35 mg	40 mg	45 mg	50 mg
Volume (mL)	(6 mL)	(7 mL)	(8 mL)	(9 mL)	(10 mL)

Administer a 60 U/kg bolus of unfractionated **heparin** IV (maximum 4000 U bolus for patients ≥70 kg followed by a 12 U/kg/hr unfractionated **heparin** IV infusion (maximum 1000 U/hr for patients >70 kg) to maintain an aPTT of 50-70 seconds.

- Consider the administration of a **GP IIb/IIIa receptor inhibitor** for patients younger than 75 with extensive anterior MIs and minimal risk of bleeding.
  - Administer **abciximab** 0.25 mg/kg IV **AND** start an **abciximab** infusion at 0.125 µg/kg/min IV

      OR
  - Administer **eptifibatide** 180 µg/kg IV **AND** start an **eptifibatide** infusion at 2 µg/kg/min IV

BOX 7-2 Checklist to Determine a Patient's Eligibility for Fibrinolytic Therapy

Initial Patient Assessment

Yes	No	
☐	☐	Pain lasting greater than 15 minutes but less than 12 hours
☐	☐	Hypertension: systolic blood pressure > 180 mm Hg
☐	☐	Diastolic blood pressure >110 mm Hg
☐	☐	Right vs. left arm systolic BP difference greater than 15 mm Hg (suspect aortic aneurysm)
☐	☐	Signs and symptoms of congestive heart failure
☐	☐	Signs and symptoms of cardiogenic shock
☐	☐	12-lead ECG with significant ST segment and T wave changes
☐	☐	Estimated time of arrival at ED _____

History

Yes	No	
☐	☐	Recent (within 6 weeks) major surgery (e.g., intracranial or intraspinal surgery), obstetrical delivery, organ biopsy, or previous puncture of noncompressible blood vessels
☐	☐	Significant head or facial trauma within previous 6 months
☐	☐	Pregnant female
☐	☐	Hemostatic defects, including those secondary to severe hepatic or renal disease, and anticoagulants.
☐	☐	CPR greater than 10 minutes
☐	☐	Any other condition in which bleeding may occur, especially if its management would be particularly difficult because of its location
☐	☐	Cerebrovascular disease, including cerebrovascular accident (CVA), seizure, cerebral aneurysm, intracranial neoplasm, or arteriovenous (AV) malformation
☐	☐	Suspected aortic dissection or known aneurysm

BOX 7-3 Contraindications and Cautions for the Use of Fibrinolytic Agents in Acute Myocardial Infarction

Absolute Contraindications

- Active internal bleeding (e.g., gastrointestinal or genitourinary); excluding menses
- Any prior intracerebral hemorrhage
- Significant closed-head or facial trauma within 3 months
- Ischemic stroke within 3 months
- Recent intracranial or intraspinal surgery or trauma
- Known intracranial neoplasm, arteriovenous malformation, or cerebral aneurysm
- Suspected aortic dissection

Relative Contraindications

- Recent puncture of noncompressible blood vessels
- Known bleeding diathesis
- For streptokinase/anistriplase: prior exposure (more than 5 days ago) or prior allergic reaction to these agents

- Traumatic or prolonged (greater than 10 minutes) CPR
- Major surgery (less than 3 weeks)
- Current use of oral anticoagulants (e.g., warfarin sodium) with INR ≥2-3
- History of recent (within 2-4 weeks) gastrointestinal, genitourinary, or other internal bleeding
- Active peptic ulcer
- History of chronic, severe, poorly controlled hypertension
- Severe uncontrolled hypertension on presentation (SBP greater than 180 mm Hg or DBP greater than 110 mm Hg)
- History of prior ischemic cerebrovascular accident greater than 3 months, dementia, or known intracranial pathology not covered in contraindictions
- Pregnancy

NOTE: If a GP IIb/IIIa receptor inhibitor is administered in combination with a fibrinolytic agent, the dosage of the fibrinolytic agent should be reduced to approximately half of that indicated above (e.g., 5-U bolus of reteplase IV initially; 15- to 25-mg bolus of tenecteplase IV).

CAUTION: After the administration of any of the above, closely monitor the patient for any bleeding.

D. Management of Congestive Heart Failure

Left Heart Failure Secondary to Left Ventricular Myocardial Infarction

Prehospital/Emergency Department

If the patient has signs and symptoms of CHF secondary to left heart failure, the result of left ventricular MI:

- Place the patient in a semi-reclining or full upright position, if possible, while reassuring the patient and loosening any tight clothing.
- Secure the airway and administer high-concentration oxygen.
- Reassess the patient's vital signs, including the respiratory and circulatory status.

- Administer **a vasodilator**, if the patient's systolic blood pressure is 100 mm Hg or greater, to reduce pulmonary congestion and edema, if not administered earlier for pain.
  - Administer **nitroglycerin** 0.4 mg by sublingual tablet or lingual aerosol, and repeat every 5-10 minutes as needed for a total of three applications

    AND

  - Start an IV infusion of **nitroglycerin** at a rate of 10-20 μg/min and increase the rate of infusion by 5-10 μg/min every 5-10 minutes until signs and symptoms of congestive heart failure improve or maximum dose of 400 μg/min is reached.

NOTE: If the mean arterial blood pressure drops below 80 mm Hg or the systolic blood pressure drops below 90 mm Hg at any time:

  - Slow or temporarily stop the IV infusion of nitroglycerin

- Institute continuous positive airway pressure (CPAP) ventilation (Box 7-4)
  - Consider the administration of a rapidly acting **diuretic** to reduce pulmonary edema if there are signs of volume overload such as significant peripheral edema.
  - Administer **furosemide** 20-40 mg (0.25-0.50 mg/kg) IV slowly over 4-5 minutes

NOTE: The role of diuretics in the treatment of acute CHF is controversial and should be guided by a determination of the patient's

BOX 7-4   Sample protocol for CPAP Administration

Continuous Positive Airway Pressure (CPAP) has been shown to rapidly improve vital signs, gas exchange, the work of breathing, decrease the sense of dyspnea, and decrease the need for endotracheal intubation in patients who suffer from shortness of breath from asthma, COPD, pulmonary edema, CHF, and pneumonia. In patients with CHF, CPAP improves hemodynamics by reducing preload and afterload.

Indications:

Any patient who is complaining of shortness of breath for reasons other than trauma and:

a. Is awake and able to follow commands
b. Is over 12 years old and is able to fit the CPAP mask
c. Has the ability to maintain an open airway (GCS > 10)
d. Has a systolic blood pressure above 90 mmHg
e. Sign and Symptoms consistent with asthma, COPD, pulmonary edema, CHF, or pneumonia

Contraindications:

1. Patient is in respiratory arrest
2. Patient is suspected of having a pneumothorax
3. Patient has a tracheostomy
4. Patient is vomiting

Precautions:

Use care if patient:

a. Has failed at past attempts at noninvasive ventilation
b. Complains of nausea or vomiting
c. Has inadequate respiratory effort

Procedure:

1. **EXPLAIN THE PROCEDURE TO THE PATIENT**
2. Ensure adequate oxygen supply to ventilation device
3. Place the patient on continuous pulse oximetry and cardiac monitoring
4. Place the delivery device over the mouth and nose and use 5 cm H20 PEEP initially and titrate as needed. Do not exceed 20 cm H20 pressure
5. Check for air leaks
7. Monitor vital signs at least every 5 minutes. CPAP can cause BP to drop. Level of consciousness is the most sensitive indicator of degree of respiratory distress
8. If respiratory status deteriorates, remove device and consider positive pressure ventilation with BVM or proceed to endotracheal intubation.

BOX 7-4 Sample protocol for CPAP Administration—cont'd

Removal Procedure:

1. CPAP therapy should be continuous and should not be removed unless the patient can not tolerate the mask or experiences respiratory failure.

Special Notes:

1. For EMS do not remove CPAP until hospital device is ready to be placed on patient.
2. Most patients will improve in 5-10 minutes. If no improvement within this time, consider intermittent positive pressure ventilation.
3. Watch patient for gastric distention. Have patient breath through nose to avoid swallowing air.
4. Use nitroglycerin infusion rather than spray to prevent dispersal on rescuers. If nitroglycerin tablets used, attempt to minimize interruptions of CPAP.
5. May be the treatment of choice in a patient with a DNR/DNI order.
6. Consider the administration of lorazepam for anxiety associated with CPAP use bearing in mind that lorazepam may result in respiratory suppression.

---

volume status in combination with renal function and the level of critical electrolytes such as sodium and potassium.

- Consider the administration of an angiotensin-converting enzyme (ACE) inhibitor;
  - Administer **captopril** 6.25-12.5 mg sublingually

E. Management of Cardiogenic Shock
Prehospital/Emergency Department

1. Assess the patient's circulatory status and vital signs, including the level of consciousness, and repeat as the situation requires and circumstances permit.

2. Administer a vasoconstrictive agent (norepinephrine) or an inotropic/vasoconstrictive agent (dopamine) as follows;
   If the systolic blood pressure is less than 70 mm Hg:
   ◦ Start an IV infusion of **norepinephrine** at an initial rate of 0.5-1.0 µg/min and adjust the rate of infusion up to 30 µg/min to increase the systolic blood pressure to 70-100 mm Hg.
   NOTE: The infusion of norepinephrine may be replaced by an infusion of dopamine at this point.

   Systolic blood pressure 70-100 mm Hg: and signs/symptoms of shock
   ◦ Start an IV infusion of **dopamine** at an initial rate of 2.5-5.0 µg/kg/min and adjust the rate of infusion up to 20 µg/kg/min to increase the cardiac output and elevate and maintain the systolic blood pressure within normal limits.

   Systolic blood pressure 70-100 mm Hg and **NO** signs/symptoms of shock
   ◦ Start an IV infusion of **dobutamine** at an initial rate of 2-5 µg/kg/min and adjust the rate of infusion up to 20 µg/kg/min to maintain systolic blood pressure within normal limits.

   NOTE: When administering vasoconstrictive agents, the systolic blood pressure must be monitored frequently so that the systolic blood pressure stays within a certain range. The rate of administration of such agents is decreased if the systolic blood pressure rises above 100 mm Hg and increased if the systolic blood pressure drops below 90 mm Hg.

Emergency Department

If cardiogenic shock continues in spite of maximal therapy, the use of a mechanical device such as an intra-aortic balloon pump to augment the vascular circulation should be considered.